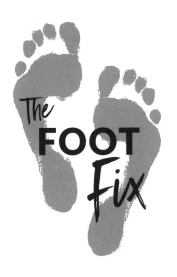

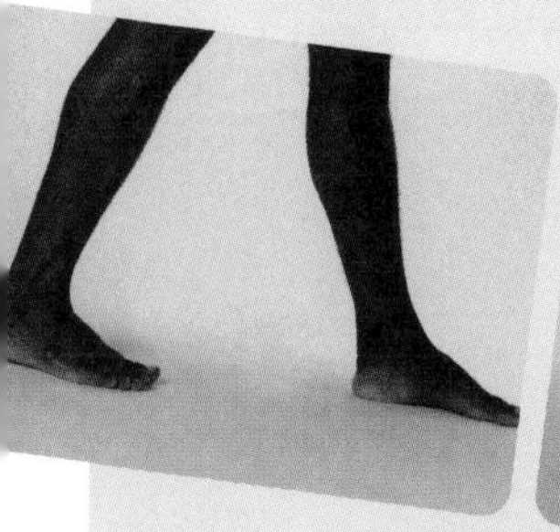
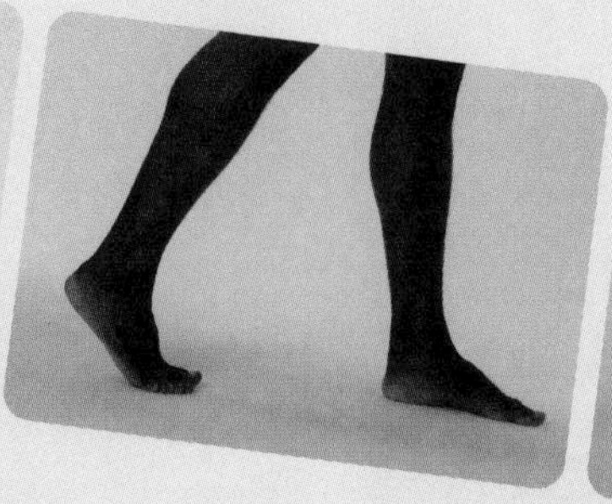
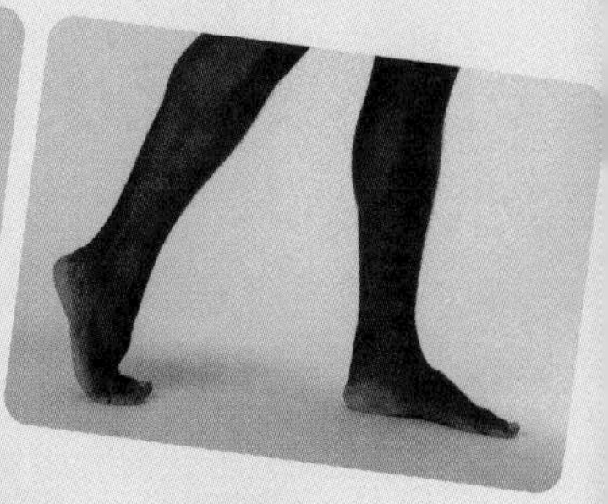
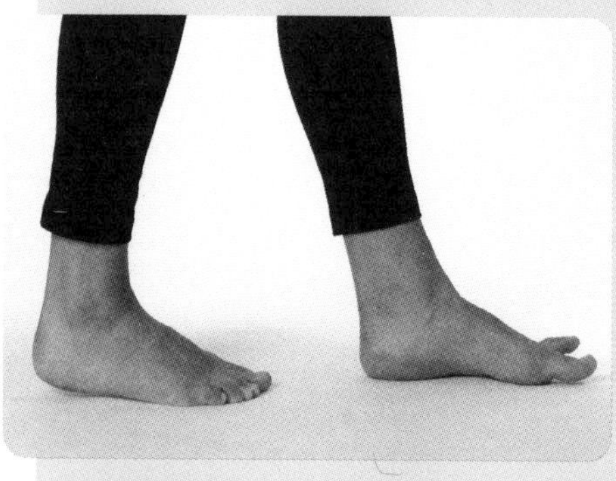
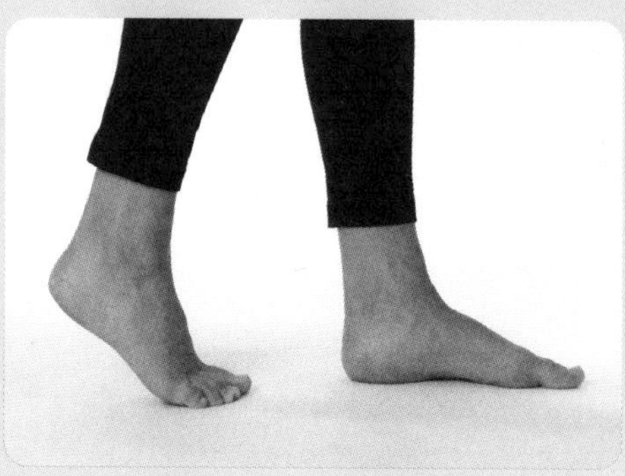
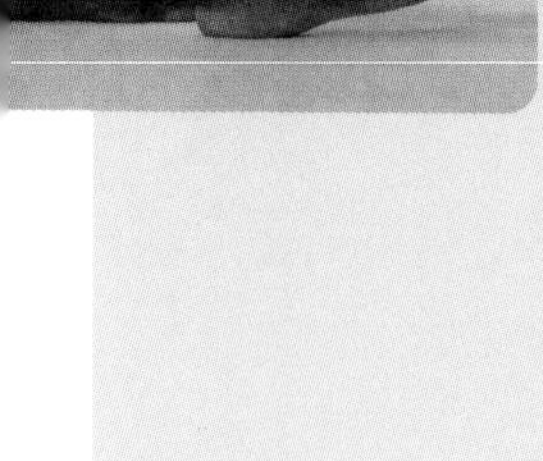

The FOOT Fix

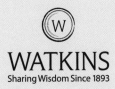

4 WEEKS TO HEALTHIER, HAPPIER FEET

Yamuna Zake

W

WATKINS
Sharing Wisdom Since 1893

The Foot Fix
Yamuna Zake
CO-WRITER: Stephanie Golden

First published in the UK and USA in 2021 by
Watkins, an imprint of Watkins Media Limited
Unit 11, Shepperton House, 83–93 Shepperton Road
London N1 3DF

enquiries@watkinspublishing.com

COMMISSIONING EDITOR: Fiona Robertson
COPYEDITOR: Becky Miles
HEAD OF DESIGN: Glen Wilkins
DESIGNER: Luise Roberts
PRODUCTION: Uzma Taj
COMMISSIONED PHOTOGRAPHY: Chae Kihn
MODELS: Lloyd Knight and Sarah Payne
COMMISSIONED ARTWORK: Luise Roberts

A CIP record for this book is available from the British Library

ISBN: 978-1-78678-453-7 (Paperback)

ISBN: 978-1-78678-474-2 (eBook)

10 9 8 7 6 5 4

Typeset in Brandon Grotesque and Black Diamond

Printed in Turkey

Publishers' note: The information in this book is not intended as a substitute for professional medical
advice and treatment. If you are pregnant or are suffering from any medical conditions or health
problems, it is recommended that you consult a medical professional before following any of the advice
or practice suggested in this book. Watkins Media Limited, or any other persons who have been involved
in working on this publication, cannot accept responsibility for any injuries or damage incurred as a result
of following the information, exercises or therapeutic techniques contained in this book.

www.watkinspublishing.com

CONTENTS

Introduction

I'm a body educator and therapist, and I'm passionate about feet. My mission in this book is to show you how to prevent and relieve foot pain yourself – and it's *easy*. Foot Fix, a four-week program I created, is simple to learn and practice because it's based on something you already do: walking.

Over 40 years of helping people relieve pain and improve their bodies, I learned that when the feet are fully functional, every other part of the body starts improving. Aches and pains that people couldn't get rid of suddenly were gone once I showed them how to properly align the parts of their feet and get each part doing its job.

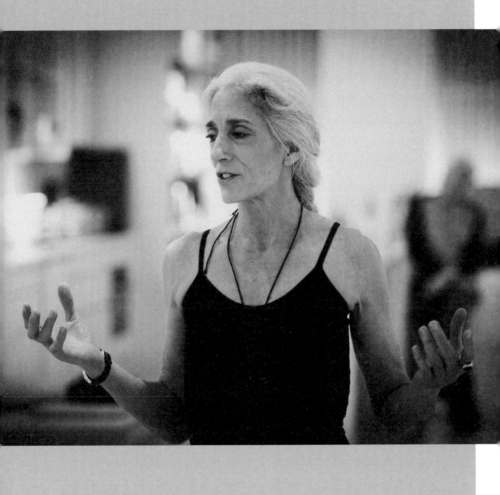

I am dedicated to demystifying the body and providing simple, powerful tools that make lifelong fitness and well-being a reality for everyone. My work had its origin in 1979, when my daughter's birth injured my left hip and I couldn't find any effective treatment. Chiropractic, acupuncture, orthopedics – nothing worked. I was a yoga teacher and wound up healing my hip myself using my yogic knowledge. Out of this experience I created Yamuna Body Logic, a hands-on therapy that became a full-time healing practice. I've treated a great range of body problems, including back pain, knee, hip and shoulder injuries, sciatica and the six foot conditions described in Chapter 4.

My original impetus for developing my foot programs was watching my mother struggle with her extremely narrow feet and their eventual aging process. She found it almost impossible to get shoes that fit, so was forced to shove her feet into shoes that cramped her toes. While I was growing up she always had hammertoes (see p.144) as a result of these ill-fitting shoes, but they didn't bother her so she never complained. It wasn't until she was in her sixties that I looked at her feet and noticed that all her toes were crossing over each other. I'd had no idea that hammertoes could become disabling, but at that point she began to lose her balance and became less and less stable walking. Realizing that I, too, could easily develop hammertoes, I began to create more and more footwork to ensure that I'd never repeat her pattern. Then, the year I hit 52, I woke up one morning, looked down, and saw that every single toe, except for my big toes, was a hammertoe. It was a shock. I was at that menopausal age when, due to hormonal changes, the bones begin to manifest rapid signs of aging, which show up quickly in the feet.

I worked on my toes and straightened them out – but the next morning they were bent again. So I realized that if I wanted to break the pattern when it was just beginning, I had to focus even more on my feet. Foot fitness became a daily practice that I continued until most of my toes stayed straight. That was over ten years ago, and my feet never became like my mother's.

This book promises that once you complete the Foot Fix program, your entire body will feel better. You will see that working on your feet can transform not only your physical body but how you think and feel. Your whole mental outlook will be brighter as you learn to stand fully on your foundation and feel supported from the ground up.

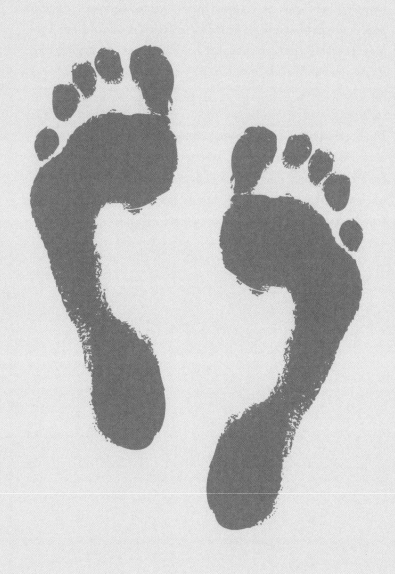

Chapter 1

Build a Foot Foundation that Supports You for Life

This chapter explains why it's so important to take care of your feet and build a solid foundation that supports you for your whole life. You'll learn how your feet may be involved in any ache or pain you have in another part of your body. Once you start paying attention to your feet, the awareness you build helps increase your awareness of the rest of your body, enhancing your wellness and helping you identify any issues at an early stage.

Barbara, a woman in her mid-fifties who came to one of my foot classes, is an inspiring example of just how fast and effective Foot Fix is.

Barbara showed up for class on a walker. A long history of severe ankle sprains had left her ankles weak, and her feet flat, so they couldn't hold her up any more. She used the walker because she was terrified of falling, and as a result was hunched way over. And being so dependent on the walker only increased her risk of falling if she tried to do without it.

The class began with a basic practice I call the Walking Test (you'll begin with it too). Since it required taking several steps across the floor, Barbara was unable to do it. She did do the second basic practice, the Power Stance, by standing and holding on to a barre. As we went on to work the four parts of the feet, she was able to do most of the routines.

Watching her, I couldn't tell whether she was really getting what I was teaching, but she was trying. At the end of the class we repeated the Walking Test, as a way to measure everyone's improvement. I was thrilled to see that though Barbara was a little shaky, she did the test without the walker and without the barre!

Afterward Barbara told me she had always thought of the foot as a single unit, but the class had made her realize it had different parts, each with its own job to do, and that she could feel and work with each part separately to teach it how to do that job. Now she knew she could get her feet stable and working again all by herself, in a simple step-by-step process. She left the class full of hope.

No matter what other parts of the body I teach about, I always come back to the feet, because they are not just our foundation, but a key to general health and well-being. In 40 years of experience, I've seen many people's lives affected by foot pain that could have been relieved or avoided in the first place if they just understood the basic concepts and practiced the easy routines that Barbara learned in that class. That's what Foot Fix will teach you, and it's the reason I wrote this book.

As you work through the program you'll learn how you developed your personal walking pattern and how to create a healthier gait. Improving your gait can relieve any foot pain, and even if you have no pain, doing this work is extremely beneficial as it can prevent you from developing foot problems in the future. You'll discover what it is to stand solidly on your feet and use them in a way that benefits both your body and your mind.

When people take their painful feet to a doctor, they get a diagnosis, say plantar fasciitis or bunion. I think of this as name-calling: they get labeled. The moment someone gets this label, they go home, get online, read up about what they "have" and all the standard treatments. But none of these treatments teaches them how it happened in the first place or suggests what they can do to heal it themselves. I tell people the bad news is that you did this to yourself – and the good news is that you can also fix it yourself, by retraining your feet to walk more correctly. All you need is a simple understanding of your feet and a step-by-step approach – information no one has ever given you before.

Foot Fix will teach you how to make each part of your feet work properly, so they don't break down in the ways that trigger those standard diagnoses. If your feet hurt, you'll learn why this happened and how to fix it without a podiatrist, orthotics, special shoes or surgery. When the four basic parts of your feet are doing their jobs (see p.36–9), they hold you up the way they're supposed to and function painlessly, as they are meant to. And you can keep them that way by practicing Foot Fix routines for only five to ten minutes a day.

Like Barbara, people in my classes easily grasp the basic concepts, and a one-hour class transforms them. They walk out standing taller, feeling more energetic and lighter on their feet. They exclaim how much better their whole body feels. As you move through the program, you too will become keenly aware of the different parts of your feet and will feel wonderful changes happening as you practice the routines.

You'll also become more aware of your feet in a mindful way. Doing the routines actually gives your feet information, and you'll know when each foot part really grasps that information, because you'll feel the difference when you stand or walk. Once you have this awareness, you'll notice when you fall back into an old misaligned foot pattern and this will alert you to mindfully shift into a healthier one.

Even if your feet feel fine right now, you are almost certainly not walking as well as you could, for two reasons: first, because you never learned how to use your feet correctly, and second, because from early childhood you have worn shoes, which change the natural shape of your feet and thereby affect your gait. Chances are that at some point your feet will start to bother you, since, as the next chapter explains, over time a poorly aligned walking pattern creates a repetitive stress pattern that will cause an injury to a part of the foot that is continually overused.

In my experience, most people wait until they're in pain before they pay attention to their feet, but since you only get one pair of them and they'll be moving you around for a lot of years, why not start taking care of them now? If you spend just 15 minutes a day over four weeks learning to get your feet fully functional, you are far less likely to develop foot problems afterwards. If you're a parent, teach the routines to your kids. The younger people start, the less chance there is of foot breakdown, pain and lost mobility in later years.

WHY HEALTHY FEET ARE CRUCIAL

As I worked on people's bodies, I discovered that even though I was able to relieve their problems, if I didn't fix their feet the problems would recur. As I developed methods to work on the feet, I found that correcting foot alignment often improved the original issue, such as hip pain, for example. It became clear to me that the feet are absolutely crucial to the well-being of the entire body. Because your feet are your foundation, they're connected to every problem you may have elsewhere in your body. No matter where an injury is, you stand on it. In fact, you can usually track it all the way down to the feet. For example, there's almost always a relationship between a knee or hip problem and the feet. If a hip or knee is not aligned properly, the foot below it will be misaligned too. Since misaligned feet don't actively hold you up, your body weight drops heavily into them, locking in the misalignment pattern that originally caused the knee or hip problem. Over time, the feet break down, causing other problems such as low back pain or tightness in your knees, hips or back. In general, if you try to fix an injured part without realigning your feet, the chances are that the injury will come back.

The converse is also true. The more function your feet have, the more strongly they support you in an upright position. Your whole body feels lighter and freer. You stand straight; your posture improves. You discover that when your feet really hold you up, it's actually hard to collapse and slump. You will feel these things are true from the moment you begin my program and take your first Power Stance (see p.63).

José's experience demonstrates this reciprocal relationship between the feet and body posture:

José was a triathlete who came to me with a pain in one hip that was preventing him from training for a marathon. I asked him to walk back and forth so I could analyze his gait and hip movement. After a few minutes of observation, I told him to take off his running shoes. When I saw his feet I knew they were the source of the hip problem. They were like a baby's feet – with very little muscle development at all.

José was extremely disciplined and trained constantly. I inquired whether he gave his feet any attention during his training sessions, and he looked at me like I was crazy.

"Do you always train with your shoes on?" I asked.

"Of course!" he said.

I explained that the long leg muscles that start at the hips run all the way down to the soles of the feet. What his running shoes did was, in effect, cut off the connection between the parts of those muscles that were in his feet and the parts in his legs and hips. So, while his leg muscles were extremely developed, there was no muscle strength or function where those same muscles ended – in his feet. I told him that running shoes were like down comforters. When you put them on, you're essentially putting your feet to sleep in a comfy, cozy bed. And that was the most likely cause of the hip problem.

José was dubious, but open to trying something new if it would get him back to training competitively. So I taught him some basic foot routines and told him to do them every day before he trained. He returned a week later, saying he didn't understand why but his hip was much better. He'd also noticed that, now he was including his feet in his training – and paying attention to his gait while running – he'd seen improvements in his speed and stride.

Working with thousands of people has shown me that most people's feet have little of the full function and movement they are designed to have. In this book you'll find all the fundamental, essential education about your feet that even today's body-conscious culture does not seem to provide.

Try This

ACTIVATE YOUR FEET, LIFT YOUR BODY

- Stand and position your bare feet parallel to each other and hip distance apart.

- Slump, dropping your shoulders, chest and head toward your hips. Stay here for a minute or two, letting your entire upper body weight collapse.

- Notice how heavy this posture makes you feel, with so much weight bearing into your feet.

- Now keep your feet in the same position but press them into the floor. Press the toes down with extra force.

- Keeping the toes pressed into the floor, inhale and lift the entire body. Feel how easy it is for the body to lift when the feet are engaged.

- Next, try using the inhalation to lift the body without pressing the feet into the floor. What happens? Do you feel your weight bearing back down into your feet?

This short, simple exercise shows what a tremendous difference active, functioning feet can make!

THE FOOT FIX PROGRAM

I designed Foot Fix for you to progress easily, step-by-step, from the heel (Week 1) to the outside edge of the foot (Week 2), to the ball of the foot (Week 3) and finally to the toes (Week 4). As you move through the program you "wake up" each part of the foot in the correct order and get it working properly again, while integrating it with the work you've done in the previous weeks.

In Week 1, you also learn the two basic practices you will use throughout the four weeks and beyond: the Walking Test (see p.58) and the Power Stance (see p.63). You use the Walking Test to find out which parts of your feet aren't actively functioning. Then each time you finish a program session, you do the test again to measure how much improvement you've created and which parts still need work. During the day, you use it to stay mindful of your feet. And you use it when you get home to remove the constricting effects of whatever shoes you've been wearing.

The Power Stance aligns your feet correctly for all the routines that follow and begins to build and strengthen your arches. You begin and end each routine by taking the Power Stance. It's also a tool to develop mindfulness of your feet, since you can do it all day, whenever you're standing, to remind your body how good it feels to stand correctly.

By the end of Week 4, you'll have an awareness of how each part of the foot functions, based on your actual experience of it. You'll know how your gait may be misaligned, which postural patterns created that misalignment, and how to create a healthy, balanced gait that will benefit your posture enormously. From then on, you'll be aware of what your feet need from day to day and can pick and choose the appropriate routines.

One reason Foot Fix is so effective is that you can't *not* feel a difference after every single routine. For example, when you take the Power Stance you're aware of your posture becoming upright. After doing the Week 1 routines you'll have a clear sensation of the full shape of your heels and can shift your weight back into them. Since the heel bones are stronger and designed to bear more weight than the balls of your feet or your toes, this shift improves your gait and posture. As you progress through the weeks, you first become aware of the separate parts of your feet, then develop strength and flexibility in each part. Feeling these changes as they happen really motivates you to continue!

Chapters 4 and 5 offer ways to extend the program. Chapter 4 describes how to relieve six common problems: bunions, plantar fasciitis, flat feet/ fallen arches, hammertoe, Morton's neuroma and hallux rigidus. For each problem, I explain what causes it, then give specific routines for fixing it as well as mindful practices to reinforce the effects of the routines.

In Chapter 5, you'll find a set of mindful practices you can do throughout the day to ensure you stay aware and keep your feet strong and healthy. And since anything you do for your feet is good, this chapter also includes some ideas for complementary treats you can give your feet.

Last, you'll find a page with information about how you can use some of my foot products to do more intensive work on your feet.

FOOT FIX BENEFITS

While the Foot Fix program will help everybody who undertakes it, certain groups of people will derive particular benefits:

- *People with a common foot problem* – plantar fasciitis, bunion, Morton's neuroma, flat feet, hammertoe or hallux rigidus. They can fix it themselves and learn to avoid getting it again.

- *Athletes* can prevent knee, hip and back injuries by ensuring that all four parts of the foot work as they should. Plus, fully functional feet will measurably improve performance.

- *Children* may have foot problems that are genetic. However, if parents make foot care a family affair, children will develop healthy walking habits and have the best chance of avoiding foot problems of all types.

- *Older adults* will be more stable and less likely to fall when their feet function properly. When the feet don't work right, neither do the leg and hip muscles, so healthy feet also improve mobility and balance.

- *Women* can wear any shoes they like – including stilettos – by using the Walking Test to work the negative effects of the shoes out of their feet.

- *Dancers* can prevent common dance injuries that can shorten careers, such as hip, knee and ankle problems.

- *People with chronic pain* are likely to have a misalignment pattern in the feet that corresponds to their pain pattern. Changing the foot pattern can help relieve the problem in the painful part.

CARING FOR YOUR FEET GOES BEYOND YOUR FEET

Foot Fix stands out from most other types of exercise because nothing you will learn here can be done by rote, as people often do when running on a treadmill, for example. That's what I mean when I say this program is mindful: you will develop an acute awareness of your body. Each time you do a routine, you will both understand *and feel* what it does for your feet, because each routine produces an immediate change. Your mind takes this in and keeps it in your memory bank because it *wants* your body to feel better.

For this reason, anything you learn as you do the routines helps focus your mindful attention on your feet during your day. You can do quite a few routines while you're standing in line, for example, and the more you do them the greater the change you'll see and feel.

Some years ago, I stood at my studio door and observed a client as she walked out. Maria had come for a foot session because of plantar fasciitis with acute pain and inflammation. By the end of the session she was overjoyed to be pain free. As I watched, she strolled down the street, talking on her phone, and by the time she reached the corner she had already fallen back into the old walking pattern that had caused the problem in the first place. I realized that her mind was not with her body; it had totally disconnected from the work we had just done. At that moment, I knew I needed to introduce mindful awareness into my treatment. People needed to learn how to pay attention, in order to understand why they have pain and then to maintain the improvements created by the Foot Fix work.

When Maria returned a week later, her plantar fasciitis was still there. This time I made sure she participated actively, both physically and mentally, in the session. I had her take the Power Stance and feel the effects. I also explained exactly why each routine would help heal her and had her pause after each routine to check in, process and understand how that routine had improved her feet. She grew excited as she began to understand which movement patterns caused her pain and which foot positions and routines immediately relieved it. She began telling me what effect each new routine had even before I asked. This was important, because now she didn't need me to tell her what had happened; she could identify it herself. She had made the mindful foot connection.

I also taught Maria how to check on her feet all day long so she could catch herself falling into the old pattern and return to the healthy one. I sent her off with homework: the Walking Test and two routines to do every day, plus an instruction to watch her foot alignment during her daily activities and correct it as necessary.

A week later she came again, thrilled at having experienced very little pain. Even better, when her feet did hurt she looked down at them, and sure enough they were back in the old alignment. She was now able to realign her feet and get herself out of pain right away. I could see in her face how empowered she felt as a result.

This mindful component of Foot Fix is as essential for success as doing the exercises. You need to make a conscious effort to stay mindful of your feet until the correct posture and gait become habitual for your body. After that, you'll continue to use your mindfulness to investigate and resolve any problems that come up.

Foot Fix is also key to what I call Body Sustainability. This term refers to proactive techniques that you can use to keep your body working happily for you in every decade of your life. The tools you learn in Foot Fix should enable you to do this for your feet. Since nonfunctioning feet affect the well-being of the entire body, fixing them improves not just your posture but also your state of mind. When the body weight drops into your feet, you feel heavy all over. But the moment you shift into the Power Stance, you feel lighter in your body, your brain works better, and you see, think and talk more clearly. Your whole you feels better!

Now that you understand why paying attention to your feet is so important and beneficial, Chapter 2 will dive deeper into understanding the structure and functions of the four parts of the foot.

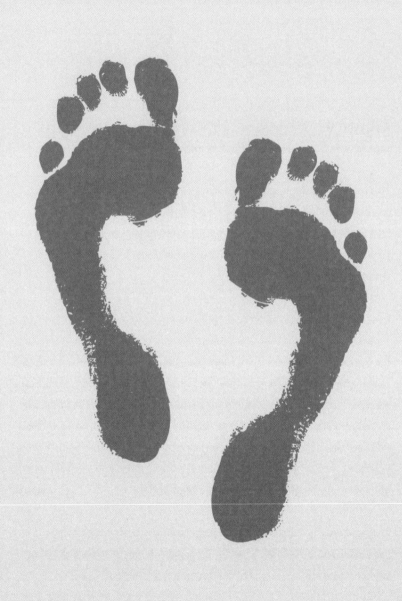

Chapter 2

Meet Your Feet

If I asked, "How do you walk?" what would you say? Could you explain exactly how your body accomplishes walking? When I first teach new students, they have no idea how to answer this question. They usually fumble for words and wind up saying something like, "I just walk!" or "It's like breathing – I just do it."

Unlike every new device you buy, the feet don't come with a user manual. When you were about a year old, you simply got up on them and started walking. Nobody told you how. Whatever walking pattern you started with got more and more engrained in your body as you grew older. And it probably included some poor habits.

Most people never think about their feet unless they become a problem. And this is precisely why most feet don't last throughout their owner's lifetime without breaking down in some way. As long as you can stand, walk and carry out your regular activities without discomfort, your poor feet will likely remain neglected and forgotten.

Often people tell me that they've never had any foot problems before, but now suddenly their feet are killing them. Shoes they've always worn are no longer comfortable, or they had to give up wearing the high heels they adored. Their feet have become too wide for their shoes, or they find themselves only buying styles with cushioned soles because their feet are so sensitive. I explain that, after all this time, their walking pattern has finally worn their feet down. Those feet are now begging for a change that will improve their gait and prevent further breakdown. Think of this book as that user manual for your feet, one that enables you to get optimal function from them.

To help you discover and correct your own pattern yourself, this chapter makes the feet really easy to understand. Once you get acquainted with the four parts of the foot and learn how to get each part working properly together with the others, your feet will do their job excellently and take you wherever you want to go.

In this chapter, I will explain how the feet are supposed to work and how they get injured. The feet are brilliantly engineered structures, designed to support your entire body weight as you move through space. When the foot bones are correctly aligned and the muscles work properly, your feet support you effortlessly. Unfortunately most people's head, shoulders and chest tend to drop forward and down because the feet are not supporting their bodies to be upright in the way active, fully functional feet should. At the same time, this collapse of the upper body puts extra pressure down into the feet, making it harder for them to maintain proper alignment.

Architecturally speaking, faulty foot alignment is like a faulty foundation of a building. Such a foundation can't sustain the structure and someday it could come tumbling down. That's what happens in the body when the feet are not the solid foundation they're meant to be.

Also, there is a big myth in our culture that people who are overweight can get rid of their foot pain if they just lose weight. I always tell people that even though excess weight can contribute to foot pain by putting more pressure into the knees and feet, once their feet are active and working properly, their foot pain will improve.

HOW YOUR FOOT BONES SUPPORT FOOT FUNCTION

Let's begin with the bones, because they rule the way a person walks. When your foot bones are correctly aligned, the foot muscles can keep your body balanced and moving. But since the feet bear all the body weight, if those bones are misaligned, the foot muscles can no longer optimally perform their function of helping move the bones. The result is an unhealthy gait, poor posture and, very likely, foot pain or discomfort somewhere down the road.

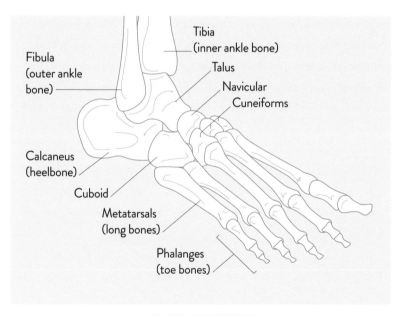

Tibia
(inner ankle bone)

Fibula
(outer ankle bone)

Talus

Navicular

Cuneiforms

Calcaneus
(heelbone)

Cuboid

Metatarsals
(long bones)

Phalanges
(toe bones)

BONES OF THE FEET

The heel bone or **calcaneus** is the main bone that you stand on. It's protected by thick padding made up of springy, bouncy cartilage, which acts as a cushion when you walk. The ankle is made up of three bones: the bottoms of the **tibia** and **fibula** (the bones of the calf) and the **talus**. The tibia and fibula rotate around the talus to bend the ankle. Just in front of the ankle are five little bones (three **cuneiforms**, the **cuboid** and the **navicular**), which form the arch. When you take a step, the ankle bends and your body weight shifts forward into these bones. There should be small movements between them to facilitate forward movement. But if the foot is not aligned correctly these bones can be forced out of place, causing dropped arches, or remain fixed as a unit, unable to move at all. Some people are told they have high arches. That means the small bones are stuck tightly together and pushed up toward the ankle, preventing the ankle from bending fully. Either way, the weight can't be smoothly transferred forward.

In front of these small bones are the five long bones (**metatarsals**) that connect to the toes. These bones do not bend, so as you step forward your weight goes from the heel to just in front of the ankle and then into the joints where the long bones connect to the toes – the area known as the ball of the foot. The ball is where the foot bends to transfer the weight forward into the toes. To facilitate this action it, too, has a great deal of padding, which helps prevent the bones from wearing out.

Four of the toes have three joints and the big toe has two. All these joints give the toes great range of movement.

Try This

ARE MY FOOT BONES ALIGNED?

- Stand barefoot in front of a mirror in your normal stance, with your feet hip width apart.

- Are the two ankle bones of each foot more or less at the same height, or is one ankle bone lower than the other?

- Is the area just in front of the ankle directly in line with the center of the ankle or does it drop inward or outward?

- Look at your toes. Is each long bone in a straight line with its toe? You can find these bones by running your finger from each toenail up the top of your foot to the ankle.

Ideally, the two ankle bones are at the same height, the small bones form an arch without dropping inward or outward, and the five long bones run straight forward and are in line with their corresponding toes. If your feet don't meet this ideal, you're in good company. It's almost impossible to find feet whose bones line up perfectly. Maybe you observed that one of your feet was well aligned and the other wasn't. If so, as you do the routines you'll be able to feel this type of difference and will know to spend a little longer working on the foot that needs better alignment.

THE LONG MUSCLES OF THE LEGS

As important as they are, your leg and foot bones couldn't move without your leg muscles. So we'll check them out next.

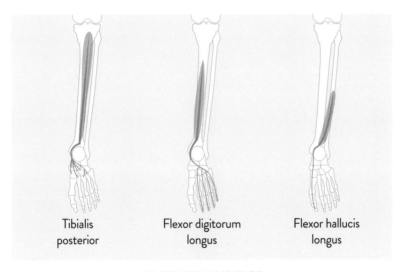

Tibialis posterior   Flexor digitorum longus   Flexor hallucis longus

BACK LEG MUSCLES

A series of long muscle chains runs from the hips down the backs of the legs, into the feet all the way to the toes. Three muscles come down the backs of the calves, turn under the edges of the feet and enter the soles just at the front of the inner heel. One of these muscles, the **tibialis posterior**, goes to five points on the little bones that make up the arch. Another, the **flexor digitorum longus**, divides into four tendons and goes out to the ends of the other four toes. The third, the **flexor hallucis longus**, goes to the end of the big toe. A misaligned gait that sends most of your weight into the inside edges of your feet will prevent these muscles from doing their job properly – the job of helping you walk and stand.

Another series of muscle chains runs down the front of the body from the hips, through the thighs and calves into the toes. Three of these muscles

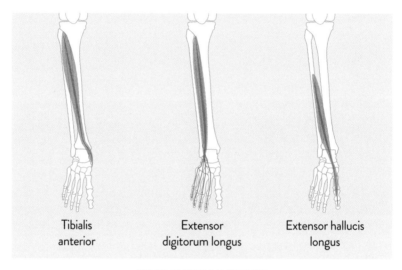

| Tibialis anterior | Extensor digitorum longus | Extensor hallucis longus |

FRONT LEG MUSCLES

run down the fronts of the calves. The **tibialis anterior** turns under the foot and goes to the base joint of the big toe. It helps maintain your foot's arch. When it's not working, all the weight goes into the big toe. The second muscle, the **extensor digitorum longus**, goes to the other four toes, and the third, the **extensor hallucis longus**, goes to the top of the big toe. These muscles help stretch the toes and ankles forward.

Both these sets of muscles – front and back – need to be equally functional in order for the feet and ankles to transfer weight properly as you walk.

There are also three important muscles – the **peroneus longus**, **peroneus brevis** and **peroneus tertius** – that run down the outside of the calf from the knee to the ankle. Their job is to support the outer foot and ankle.

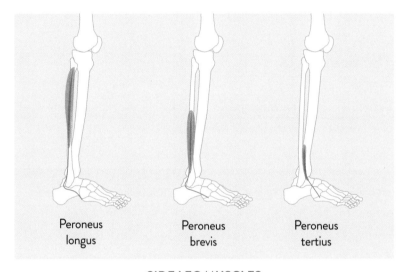

Peroneus
longus

Peroneus
brevis

Peroneus
tertius

SIDE LEG MUSCLES

When they're working well, they keep the weight on the outside edges of the feet where it should be. If they aren't working well, the weight bears into the inner side of the foot, and can break the arch down. Throughout the four weeks of the Foot Fix program, you'll be activating these muscles and getting them to work as they should.

THE FOUR PARTS OF THE FOOT AND HOW THEY WORK

Anatomy textbooks describe the foot as having three parts, but for the practical purpose of teaching people to correct their gait, I divide it into four: heel, outside edge, ball of the foot and toes.

The heel

Everyone knows where their heel is. But whether they know how to stand on it correctly may be quite a different story.

The heel functions like a launch pad: bearing weight into it gives you the momentum you need to transfer your weight forward through all four parts of the foot, one after the other, as you walk. It's the largest bone in the foot, made to support your entire body weight, so it makes sense that it should bear the most weight when you stand. The moment you stand with your weight bearing into your heels, your whole back will feel relaxed – as though you're now standing the way you're supposed to – and you'll realize that the entire back of your body is connected to your heels.

However, years of shoe-wearing have frozen most people's feet into a single unit, so they tend to stand with their weight shifted forward into the balls of the feet where the bones are not as strong or stable. This is a very common standing position and it causes the toes, thighs and lower back to tense up and grip, which creates unnecessary tension in the body.

By contrast, when your weight is in the heels, you stand straighter and your body feels lighter. This is why the first focus in the Foot Fix program is to wake up your heels, free them from being stuck to the front parts of the foot, and restore their function. By "wake up," I mean stimulate them to make you aware of them in a way you haven't been before. Once you fully *feel* your heels, you naturally shift your weight backward into them. Your body will stand more upright and feel more solid, and you will no longer put extra stress into the balls of the feet and toes.

The outside edge

The outside edge of your foot includes the outer side of the heel, the two outer long bones and the outer edge of the ball of the foot where these two bones attach to the two outer toes. The outer edge also has padding that cushions it as it transfers weight to the ball of the foot.

Over years of observing thousands of feet, I discovered that most people never use the outside edges of their feet when they walk. Instead, they walk mostly on the inner side of their feet, and the outer part works very little or not at all. When the entire outer side does nothing as you walk, all your body weight goes only into the inner side of the foot, which is not built to take this amount of weight. The inner ball of the foot and the big and second toes are overused and, chances are, over time the foot will suffer from this repetitive weight-bearing.

And because the outer edge is not actively supporting the weight bearing into it, the padding underneath it tends to "ooze" out to the side.

Once you have activated the outer edge of your foot, it can work together with the other three parts to distribute your weight over the entire foot, relieving the stress on the inner side. Standing more firmly on the outer edge will help you be more upright and you'll step forward into each stride from a strong stance.

The ball of the foot

The ball of the foot is the point where weight is transferred from the long bones into the toes. There should be a full bend between each toe and its corresponding long bone when this happens. You don't want some toes to bend fully and some not or there will be an imbalance in your gait. You should also be able to transfer your weight back and forth from one side of the ball of the foot to the other.

Unfortunately, most people's foot joints have lost their flexibility due to being stuck in shoes all day and never being stretched. These joints then become immoveable, and over time can calcify (harden) and become arthritic.

The ball of the foot has thick padding because it bears so much weight as it bends to transfer the weight forward. If there were no padding, the bones would likely wear out. (And the padding certainly comes in handy when you wear high heels, because without it you'd be standing directly on the bones.) As it is, when people walk for years with their weight shifted forward into the ball, the padding gets pushed forward and no longer properly protects this area. Often, too, when someone's weight collapses forward into their feet, the padding is displaced sideways and stops supporting the ball adequately.

The toes

Your toes are essential for both walking and standing. In fact, you'd have no balance without them. When you press your toes into the floor as you stand, you immediately feel your posture lift (see Try This on p.40). When the toes lack strength or function, they can't help support the body to be upright.

The toes' flexibility enables the foot to roll through them during the final part of each stride. As the back heel lifts to step forward, it rolls the weight through the ball of the foot into the toes. The toes of both feet press into the floor as the back foot steps forward. The foot lifts, then the heel comes down, followed by the ball of the foot, as the toes reach forward and come down last.

To fully perform these actions, the toes must be able to bend at each joint and have the strength to support the foot in its forward movement. But when we cramp them into shoes, they lose not only their correct alignment but even the memory of how to function properly.

Try This

ACTIVATE YOUR TOES

- Stand with your feet parallel, hip width apart. Shift your weight forward toward the fronts of your feet but lift your toes off the floor slightly, so they are touching it but not being used.

- Now press all ten toes into the floor as strongly as you can. What happens?

Did you find that when you aren't using your toes, you have hardly any balance? You could easily be pushed over. The moment you press them strongly into the floor, your balance improves tremendously, your stance is more upright, and your arch and general foot alignment are also better. Your feet can't support your body's weight to the best of their ability unless the toes are engaged. This is one reason that older adults whose toes have lost their ability to function properly are more likely to fall.

WATCHING YOUR STEP

Your gait is simply the way you walk. People generally grow into their gait through a variety of influences. Children watch and copy the gait of their parents or other people close to them until they encounter other influences, such as early dance training or any type of sport. An injury may cause someone to limp or otherwise compensate as the body figures out a way to walk to avoid exacerbating the injury. This imbalanced gait soon becomes the person's new normal.

Posture, gait and the way people carry themselves say a great deal about how they move through life. If your body collapses into your feet as you walk, your energy drops too and your gait becomes heavy and lethargic. By contrast, a gait that uses every part of your feet is more upbeat. It puts bounce back into the entire body, creating an overall sense of well-being.

The ideal gait

A correct gait uses all four parts of the foot. Starting from the center heel, then shifting to the outside edge of the heel, the weight transfers along the outside edge of the foot, then rolls through the ball of the foot from the little toe to the big toe. Training your feet to use the whole ball of the foot in this way will prevent you from putting extra stress into one spot. Stressing one area of the foot over a long period leads to a repetitive stress injury.

People walk in many different ways, but the misaligned gaits described below are quite common. You may recognize your own style of walking in one of them. All of these gaits may cause the bones to lose correct alignment and, as a result, the foot spreads out. You see this commonly in older people, whose feet become wider and wider. Their misaligned bones and muscles are no longer properly supporting their feet.

Misaligned gait 1: heel to big toe

In this gait, the weight goes directly from the heel to the big toe, and the person pushes off from only the big toe instead of using all five toes. As a result, the big toe becomes permanently bent toward the other toes and the knees turn in toward each other. The body weight bears into the inner sides of the legs and ankles, and the inner side of the foot hits the floor without bending or using its muscles. The bones don't shift to assist forward movement. This can cause the inner ankles to collapse and the arches to drop. This misalignment is generally called a pronated foot, but I call it a collapsed foot, because the inner ankle and the arch drop inward. It is very common among women and slowly breaks down the arches, ankles and knees.

Misaligned gait 2: slapping the whole foot down

Here the person lifts a foot to bring it forward without bending it, then slaps the entire foot down at once. Usually, the feet are slightly turned out. These feet have forgotten that they have the ability to transfer weight sequentially through the entire foot. They just move the body forward without giving it any sensation of ease of movement or uplift. The body weight usually drops into the pelvis and hips, and can cause hip or lower back problems, since with each step the weight of the whole side bears down into that side's hip and lower back.

Misaligned gait 3: shuffling

A shuffler slides one foot forward, then the other, so the feet hardly come off the floor. Like people who slap their feet down, shufflers barely use their feet. Instead of the feet being active and propelling the stride, the hips initiate the movement and the feet just come along. This provides no lift for the body. The weight drops into the feet, which can't really support the body as they should and tend to be unstable. You see this gait in older people whose feet have lost most of their ability to move due to arthritic bones and stiff muscles. Their feet have so little function that they fear losing balance, and shuffling feels more secure. Yet, it's actually the shuffling that makes it easy to lose balance and fall forward. This accident is a common result when a shoe gets stuck on a carpet and the shuffler tips over.

Misaligned gait 4: "inside walking"

In the gait I call "inside walking", the person shifts their weight from the inner heel to the big toe. As in the heel-to-big-toe gait, all the weight goes into the inner thighs, knees, calves, ankles, inside edges of the feet and big toes. This gait weakens the arch, breaks down the plantar fascia (the strong ligament between the heel and ball of the foot that becomes inflamed in plantar fasciitis) and prevents any other part of the foot from working properly. Inside walking also causes the body to collapse into the pelvis, inner thighs and knees. It prevents you from standing fully upright. If you have been told you are a pronator, you may be walking this way.

Try This

AM I DOING "INSIDE WALKING"?

In front of a mirror, take your normal standing position. Where is your weight bearing into your feet? Are your inner ankles dropping towards the floor? Are your arches dropped? Does all the weight go into your big toes? If you said yes to any of these questions, you're doing inside walking.

When you really see your ankles and feet collapsing inward, your mind will tell you it doesn't feel right. Sometimes people tell me they feel sort of silly when they perceive this, and they wonder why they do it and why they've never noticed before. But you're now aware of it – which means you can correct it!

A PLEA TO PARENTS

Instead of waiting until your children develop unhealthy walking patterns, why not begin teaching them a healthy gait as soon as they start to walk? My ideal vision would be to introduce healthy foot education in elementary school to help prevent children from developing foot, knee, hip and back problems when they grow older. But don't wait for that vision to become reality! Start training your children right now, so they never develop unhealthy walking patterns that have to be corrected later. Use everything you learn from this book with them. Make foot care a family project. If your children see you doing your Foot Fix routines, they'll want to copy you.

As I've already said, one factor in how children develop their gait is imitating their parents, so if you correct your own gait when your children are young, chances are they'll mimic you and may not need any correction themselves!

SHOES: WHERE THE PROBLEMS BEGIN

Your feet are the only part of you that's squashed all day into a form that's not their natural shape. And all day, your entire body weight bears into these constricted feet. *All* kinds of shoes, even "comfort shoes" and shoes specially designed to relieve pain, alter the natural form of your feet. It's no surprise that, starting from childhood, your feet lose parts of their function. This is why you need to teach them how to work properly again.

Shoes are stressful for the body as well as the feet. Constricting the feet in shoes gradually shortens all the muscles that run from the feet up through the legs. Eventually, this shortening restricts movement of the joints above the feet. This is why many older people lose their youthful bounce and elastic stride and may struggle just to walk down the street.

Shoes also prevent your toes from doing their best job of helping you walk correctly. Fashion dictates shapes for women's shoes that cramp the toes in a narrow space that keeps them from moving freely. Over time, the toes lose their natural straight shape. They curve, curl under, become twisted and push into other toes. Eventually, they become frozen into these unnatural positions and are cut off from their connections to the other muscles that move your legs, losing circulation, strength and the ability to function properly.

Men's shoes tend to be wider than women's, so their feet and especially their toes have more space to move. Still, many lace-up business shoes keep the foot pretty much locked into a flat position and unable to bend. After years of wearing these shoes, the foot muscles can lose their strength, the arches collapse and the feet contract into this position. This is one reason why older men can get severe leg cramps that wake them up in the middle of the night.

I used to think that there were many fewer foot problems in cultures where people often go barefoot. But when I looked into this I discovered that while these people's toes were straighter and had much better function, many had collapsed arches, flat feet and dropped inner ankles. I also saw many with the classic one-foot-turned-out-more-than-the-other habitual stance, which usually indicates a misalignment that weakens the hip, and I observed many of the common gait patterns I see in shoe wearers. My conclusion is that although most of our culture's foot problems come from wearing shoes, even if we went barefoot we would still need foot education.

So, I'm not telling you to stop wearing shoes! In fact the opposite is true. The Walking Test (see p.58) enables you to wear any shoes you like – even stilettos – without hurting your feet, as long as you do the practice once you take them off to "walk your shoes out of your feet", as I like to say. Since your feet take on the shape of whatever shoes you wear, just taking them off does not get those shoes out of your feet. But the Walking Test uncramps the foot muscles and frees them to work again.

I tell people to use the Walking Test this way all the time, and they laugh at me. But when women have been wearing tight stilettos for hours, it occurs to them to try it, and they report back that I was right. They had expected their feet to hurt the next morning but discovered that in fact they were fine!

Are there "healthier" shoes?

When I was growing up, if you were a good parent you put your children in sturdy lace-up shoes made of stiff leather with metal along the sides of the heel and sole. The idea was that the feet needed this support to develop in a healthy way. My mother made me wear these shoes, and I hated them. When the penny loafer came into style everyone else wore them and she wouldn't let me get a pair. Today's parents are advised to buy a shoe that's supportive but has a flexible sole and a wider toe bed to allow the feet to move. Beliefs about what's good for the feet keep changing. But once you've learned from the Foot Fix program how best to take care of your feet, it won't matter what the latest word about foot care turns out to be.

Many shoes for adults are marketed with the promise that they will relieve a specific foot problem. Some are said to be for people who pronate. Some have a wider toe bed or are super cushioned for sensitive feet. Others claim to mimic a natural barefoot gait. And you can buy arch supports to insert in your shoes.

What I tell people who ask me to recommend a healthy shoe is that if you know how to keep your feet working correctly, it doesn't really matter which shoe you buy. You can wear any shoes you like and your feet will stay healthy (as long as you take care of them, including doing the

Walking Test after wearing those shoes). It is never a good idea to believe that a shoe or an arch support will fix any foot problems, though they may give you a temporary fix. I also suggest that you wear a mix of different styles so your feet don't get stuck in the shape of any one style.

That said, it's wise to have a basic pair that are really comfortable to walk in as your everyday knock-around shoes. These shoes should have a completely flexible sole and a wide toe bed that lets your toes move. They should give your feet the space they need to move freely while also supporting the back, sides and front of the foot. Make sure the shoe moves with you as your feet bend to transfer weight through all four parts. This style should be the walking shoe that enables you to keep mindfully checking in with your feet throughout the day.

Now you understand how beautifully the feet are designed to support your entire weight, and why they can get injured. You've perhaps also identified your own gait, and you've become familiar with the foot bones, muscles and the four parts of the feet. You're now ready to start the Foot Fix program!

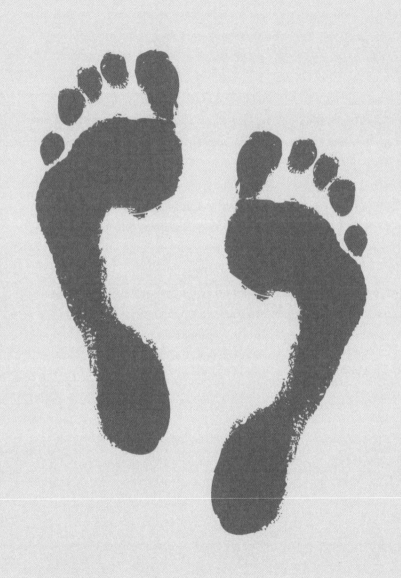

Chapter 3

The Foot Fix Program

GETTING THE MOST OUT OF FOOT FIX

You will achieve tangible results from day one of starting the Foot Fix program. The very first time you try the Walking Test and the Power Stance, you'll gain a whole new awareness of what your feet can do. As you rebuild them step-by-step, you'll feel them change with every routine and know exactly how each routine is benefiting you. And when your feet are healthier, your whole body feels better. After just one session you will be breathing more deeply, holding your body more upright, experiencing a lift in your energy and feeling lighter on your feet.

Over years of teaching I've seen that most people have no real connection to their feet – they don't know how their feet move and don't even really feel them, unless they hurt. Foot Fix is designed to change this. Using the Walking Test at the beginning and end of each session will help you really understand how your feet work and will encourage you to use them differently. It is also a simple but effective tool to measure your progress – you'll see how each routine creates new improvements, and you'll discover abilities you never dreamed of.

Often a therapeutic exercise regimen feels like a chore. It takes a long time to produce results, and the exercises can be boring. But with Foot Fix, it takes only five minutes to feel a major change. And because all the routines require you to be mindfully connected to your body, rather than simply doing repetitions by rote, it's not boring at all. As you move through the four-week Foot Fix program, each week adds another component to rebuilding your feet and gets you more in touch with a part of your body you probably never had a relationship with before.

The order of the weeks is important

You might be tempted to skip ahead to the parts of your feet you feel need help the most, but the order of the routines in the program follows the natural order of how the foot is meant to move, from the heel toward the toes. Each part needs to learn how to work in that order, so each week of the program builds on the previous week. Once you've completed the program and feel comfortable with the routines, you'll know which ones your feet need the most and can return to focus on those.

Track your progress

Consider tracking your progress in a journal. Record how each routine affects your feet, including the differences you notice between the two feet when you return to the Power Stance after each routine. Also record the improvements you achieve in each session as measured by the Walking Test.

Ask yourself the following questions to help develop greater awareness of your feet and entire body. This will help you realize just how much improvement you can feel and see.

• What sensations did you feel in the foot you worked on and in the rest of your body?

• What changes did you notice in your feet overall?

• How has your weightbearing shifted?

• How has the routine affected your posture?

• Does any other part of your body where you had some discomfort now feel better?

• Were any other parts of your body affected?

General guidelines for the four weeks and beyond

- Do all the routines barefoot.

- Throughout the program, try to stay mindful of the routines you're doing that week as you go about your day. See how often you can add in one of them whenever you're walking or standing.

- There is no need to spend more than 15 minutes on any session. However, do give yourself this amount of time to practice while you're still learning. Once you know how to activate each part of your feet, you should be able to keep them healthy with a daily practice of just five to ten minutes.

- Some routines have both sitting and standing versions. Learn to do both. If you sit much of the day at work, you can use some of that time to do seated routines. The standing routines put more body weight into the feet, which gives you better, quicker results. But if you're more likely to find the time to do the seated ones, do those. I do seated routines often, because when I'm sitting I think: why should I be doing nothing all this time?

When you complete the program, write down which routine(s) from each week feel most effective. These will be the routines you work with most of the time thereafter, together with the Walking Test and the Power Stance. When your body has become used to this work, you will only need a short daily practice to keep all the parts of your feet activated and working as they should. If you had foot pain, you'll know how to avoid the poorly aligned walking pattern that caused it and which routines keep your feet strong.

You may sometimes feel the need to work on a specific part of your feet. If so, choose routines that target those areas. If you have one of the specific foot problems listed in Chapter 4, follow the instructions there for healing that problem.

The big changes you'll feel from doing the Power Stance alone make getting started easy, and the improvements you'll see in each session as you work through Foot Fix will keep you positive and focused throughout the four weeks.

Here's to your success in getting your feet healthy and pain-free!

WEEK 1:

CREATE YOUR ARCHES, STAND ON YOUR HEELS

Week 1 starts off with the two basic exercises – the Walking Test and the Power Stance – and this is when you will discover where your arches actually come from and how easy it is to build them yourself. No arch supports needed!

The Walking Test and Power Stance are the two most important practices for your feet. They'll stay with you as a solid foundation for the routines you learn in the remaining weeks, and you'll continue using them after you complete the Foot Fix program. They're an effortless way to stay mindful and connected to your feet, anywhere and any time.

In Week 1, you will also learn the routines for the heels, the first of the four parts of the feet. These will get you standing solidly on your heels, so your weight stays in the back of your body and you start every step with good posture, instead of leading with your chest and head as so many people do. Once you've activated your heels, they'll remember their job, which is to initiate movement through the rest of the foot: the beginning of a balanced, healthy, energetic and pain-free stride.

WEEK 1 GUIDELINES

• DAYS 1–2

Start this first week with two full 15-minute sessions of practicing just the Walking Test (see p.58) and the Power Stance (see p.63). They seem simple, but since your feet were never actually taught how to walk or stand, these practices are a big lesson for them. You need to put dedicated mental and physical attention into training your feet to do them.

• DAYS 3–4

On Day 3, add the first heel routine – Waking up the Heels (see p.69) – to the Walking Test and the Power Stance. Practice all three, spending five minutes on each, for two days.

• DAYS 5–6

On Day 5, add the second heel routine – Heel-Ball-Toes (see p.73) – and practice all four for two days.

• DAY 7

Add the third heel routine – Weight-shifting (see p.75) – and practice all five routines together.

The Walking Test

This key practice is used as a test to find out which parts of your feet aren't working for you yet, then to measure your success after each practice session and ensure that your feet are absorbing the new concepts they're learning.

It also promotes mindfulness because you simply can't do it while thinking about something else. You have to be totally there. People in my classes sometimes focus so intensely on this test that they actually stop breathing and I have to remind them to take a breath!

Use the Walking Test every day to measure the changes as you work through the four weeks. You may be surprised to discover that it's quite difficult to walk through your whole foot. But even if you can't do it correctly at first, you'll become aware that your feet have the *potential* to move this way. And that's a big part of fixing foot pain.

TIP If it seems like a chore to think about how you walk all the time, remember that your goal is to learn to be present when walking. If you do the Walking Test for just one to two minutes a day, in time it will become second nature to you.

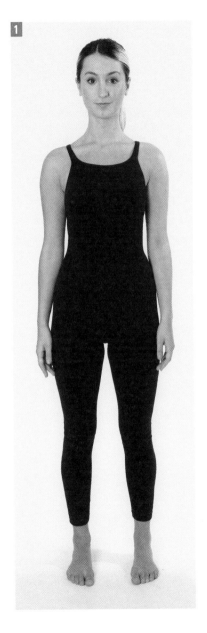

1. Stand with your feet parallel. Step one foot forward and place the center of the back of the heel on the floor.

2. Shift your weight to the *outer edge* of the *heel*. Bend your knee a little on this leg and press your weight down into that outer heel. As you press, try to stretch the entire outer edge out from the heel, all the way through the ball of the foot. You might not feel this stretch at first, but imagine it happening, and it will come. Before long you'll find that foot is stretching forward.

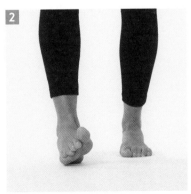

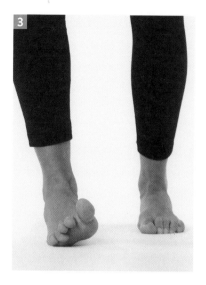

3. Keeping the weight on the outside, place the entire outside edge, from the front of the heel to the ball, down on the floor. The goal here is simply to see whether you can do this. Often people don't use the outside edge of their foot at all, and they discover they can't put weight into it or feel the pressure being exerted. Some people even lose their balance when first doing this, so take care.

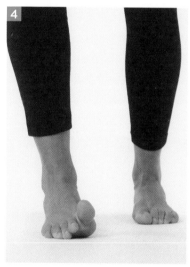

4. With the outside edge still stretched out, try to stretch the little toe and press it into the floor. Now do the same with the fourth, third, second and big toes. Your knee *must* stay over the center of your ankle, so the weight never drops inward and the ankle stays straight. You may find that three toes come down as a group, or the big toe comes down first. This shows you that you can't separate the toes or really press them into the floor – which means that you don't have full use of them. Eventually, they'll all work separately.

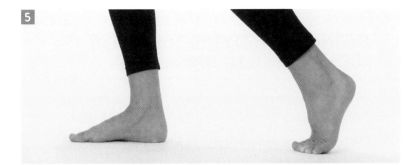

5. When you have all five toes pressing into the floor as best you can, lift the heel of your other foot, roll through the entire ball of that foot into the toes and then lift and bring that foot forward. Place the heel down first, then the outside of the foot, then the toes, one by one, as you did with the first foot. When the second foot is firmly on the floor to stabilize you, lift the heel of the first foot again and repeat the exercise. Take four or five steps with each foot this way.

6. Now compare the performances of your two feet. The first time you do this, you may find some surprising differences. Perhaps you could put your toes down separately with one foot, but the ball and toes of the other flopped down as one unit. Maybe you couldn't roll through the entire ball of the foot into the toes on one side but you could on the other. Or you could press all five toes of one foot down, while the toes of the other had no strength to press.

This information tells you which parts of each foot are functioning well and which aren't, so you know what you need to work on.

USING THE WALKING TEST AFTER COMPLETING THE PROGRAM

I urge you to make the Walking Test part of your daily life. Start your day with a few Walking Test steps. You only need to take five or six steps with each foot to get a good readout on how your feet are. Then, during the day whenever you wear flexible shoes that give your toes room to move, you can practice being mindful of your gait as you walk down the street. (This is a great routine by itself, since it gets you using your leg muscles more fully, from hips to toes.)

At the end of the day, when your feet feel tired, use the Walking Test to activate all four parts and to walk your shoes out of your feet.

The Power Stance

The Power Stance is designed to build your arches and align your feet. It is your starting position for every routine in the program: standing with feet parallel and your weight bearing into their outside edges. This stance aligns your feet correctly and begins to develop strength in your arches. Like the Walking Test, it helps you develop mindfulness, because it makes sense to your body, which feels much stronger and more grounded, yet with a great lightness and uplift. The mind and feet say yes to this wonderful feeling and want to continue creating it.

Practice the Power Stance throughout Week 1. Your goal is to get it engrained in your feet and your brain so that this new foot alignment becomes your habitual stance after you finish the program.

The Power Stance begins creating your arch simply by making a straight line with the outside edge of your foot. You can feel your arch lift just by doing it. But to fully develop and maintain healthy arches you also need the routines in Weeks 2–4 to strengthen the other parts of your feet.

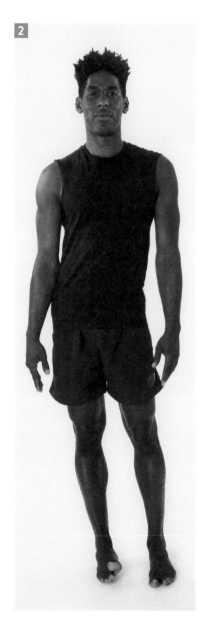

2

1. Stand with your feet parallel and hip-width apart.

2. Shift your weight into one foot. Line up the outside edge of the foot so it forms a completely straight line, from the heel to the little toe. Ideally you can line it up along the edge of a rug, tile or plank in the floor. If any padding from under the foot sticks out to the side, tilt the foot onto the outside edge, bear weight into it, and press outward with your leg and foot to tuck the padding back under the foot where it belongs. The padding is supposed to be underneath the foot. It acts as a cushion and springboard. When it oozes out to the side, it's not doing these jobs. When you look down, this foot should now look very different from the other foot, and you should feel that you're standing straighter and the padding is actually supporting you.

3. Move your hip farther out to the side so your weight goes even more into that foot, and all the toes except the fifth toe (the pinky) come off the floor. You want to feel your body weight bearing into the bones of the outer edge of the foot, outer knee, and hip. As you stay in the stance, you can feel the sensation of your weight in those bones.

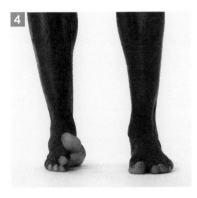

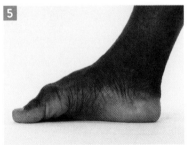

4. With your weight still going into the outside edge of the foot, lower your fourth, third, second and big toes one at a time, as best you can. (The toes are numbered 1–5, with 1 being the big toe and 5 the pinky toe.) Make sure you keep the knee directly over the middle of your foot and ankle as you do this.

5. Once all five toes are on the floor, press them down. Look: you've got an arch!

Don't worry if you can't move each toe by itself or get your second toe or big toe easily to the floor. This just indicates that you still have work to do to create length through each part of the foot. Once you retrain all the parts of your feet through the four-week program, you'll be able to do these actions.

6. Now shift your weight to the other foot and repeat steps 2–5, without losing the new stance of the first foot.

7. Once you've placed each toe of the second foot down, shift back to standing with equal weight on both feet. Make sure your weight goes into the outside edge of each foot and that all five toes are pressing into the floor.

8. Stand this way for a few moments. Take a few deep breaths and feel how your breath moves up through your body more easily, creating a sensation of uplift.

In the following weeks you'll do more specific routines to strengthen the arch and enable you to transfer weight through each part of your foot as you walk. This will help you avoid putting repetitive stress on any one part of the foot.

FEEL THE EFFECTS

- Do you feel lighter on your feet?

- Are you standing taller?

- If there was any weakness or discomfort in your lower back, is it still there?

USING THE POWER STANCE AFTER COMPLETING THE PROGRAM

The Power Stance is the quickest way to bring your feet to attention throughout the day, for example when you're standing in the kitchen chopping vegetables. Once you're in this stance, your body registers it as a smarter position to be in because it now feels effortless to stand.

The minute you catch yourself falling back into your old pattern, you can slip back into the Power Stance and immediately feel better. This is a very strong motivator! Say you're waiting for a train and learn there's going to be a delay. The normal response is for your posture to collapse. Your whole body drops, you lose your energy, you feel terrible. That doesn't serve you well. Instead, shift into the Power Stance. The moment you're upright, you realize you don't have to feel lousy. It's a posture that really helps you stay positive.

The Heels

After teaching the heel routines to a class, I asked what changes people were feeling. One woman said she could feel the entire shape of her heels for the first time. She had never experienced herself really standing on them, and now that she did, she noticed that her whole body had shifted slightly backward, which made her lower back relax completely. She was deeply impressed that just by stimulating her heels she had improved her posture, released tension in her lower back and created a sensation of lightness all through her torso. I explained that this heel work creates what shoe marketers call a "negative heel," whereby the heel is designed

Try This

WHERE'S MY WEIGHT?

Stand with your feet parallel, hip-width apart. Where's your weight? If you're like most people, most of it is going into the balls of your feet and your toes. Now consciously shift your weight back into your heels. What happens? The front of the body feels lighter and there's less pressure in your back. You're standing taller. The balls and toes are relaxed, ready for the back foot to transfer weight into them.

to be lower than the rest of the shoe, encouraging the wearer to shift the weight back into their heels before they then transfer the weight forward through the foot when walking.

As I told the class, by following my heel exercises they were creating their own negative heels. They didn't need a specially designed shoe to do this. And as you follow the heel routines described below you will soon have the same experience.

Routine 1: Waking up the Heels

This routine unglues your heels from the rest of your foot and lets you really experience what it is to stand on them fully. In just seconds, you can actually feel them holding you more upright. The seated version is great to do at your desk at work, but the standing version puts even more weight into your heels, so you can wake them up more quickly and fully.

Standing Version

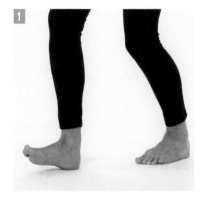

1. Stand in the Power Stance and lift one foot forward. Press it down on just the heel as though you're trying to grind it into the floor. Then press just the back of the heel into the floor, and then each side of the heel.

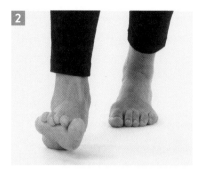

2. Try making circles with your heel as you press it into the floor, rolling it clockwise and then counterclockwise.

3. Return to the Power Stance and feel the effects.

4. Repeat with the other foot. This will most likely be a different experience as our two feet never work quite the same.

> **TIP** This routine is almost always more difficult on one side than on the other. Even if you feel you aren't doing it as well on one side, don't worry, it's still effective. We always have one dominant side, which is tighter than the other.

Seated Version

1. Sit in a chair and slide yourself toward the front of the seat. Place both feet parallel on the floor and in line with your knees.

2. Bring one foot slightly in front of the other. Lift the front of that foot so only the back of the heel is on the floor. Lean your upper body forward to provide extra force and press the back of the heel into the floor.

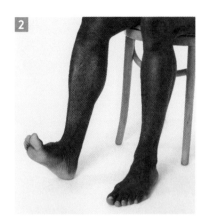

3. Keep the toes lifted and press forward through *just the heel* as far as you can – the toes and ball of your foot will come down very lightly. Lift the toes and ball and come back to your starting point, then press forward again. Repeat five times.

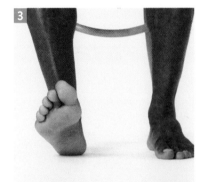

4. Turn your heel so the outer back heel presses into the floor and press it forward and backward five times.

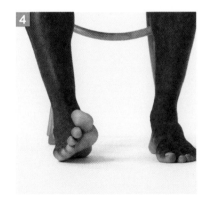

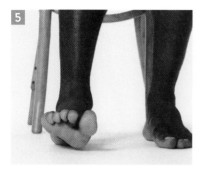

5. Turn your heel so the inside edge of the back of the heel presses into the floor and press it forward and backward five times.

6. Press the center of the heel down. Roll it in circles in one direction and then the other, several times in each direction.

7. Stand up, take the Power Stance and notice what effects you feel.

8. Repeat with the other heel.

FEEL THE EFFECTS

- Are you now more aware of the full shape of your heels?

- Is your weight bearing more into the heels and the back of your body?

- Does the front of your body feel lighter and more upright?

Routine 2: Heel-Ball-Toes

Now let's train your feet to transfer weight from the heels to the balls of the feet and the toes. Once your heels are activated, you use them as your foundation to practice rolling through the whole foot.

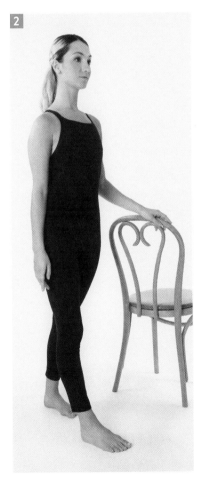

1. Hold onto a table or chair for balance if you need to.

2. Stand in the Power Stance and step one foot forward.

3. Lift the fronts of both feet so the weight goes into the heels. Bend both knees slightly and lean more into the heel of the back foot.

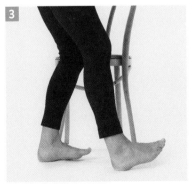

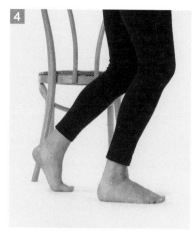

4. Keeping the knees bent, shift your weight forward into the balls of the feet and toes. Your weight moves into the front foot and the back-foot heel comes up.

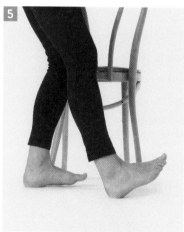

5. Shift the weight backward, rolling through the ball of the back foot and to the heels. The weight returns to the back foot, with the ball and toes of both feet off the floor. Only the back of the front heel is on the floor.

6. Repeat steps 2–5 five times with the same foot forward, then switch foot positions and repeat the entire routine.

7. Stand in the Power Stance and feel the effects.

FEEL THE EFFECTS

• Are you standing more upright?

• Is your weight going more into a point slightly in front of your heels? This is the neutral point where the body is most relaxed because it doesn't need to tense any muscles to stand erect.

• Is there less weight into your toes and balls of the feet?

• Is the front of your body lifting up out of your hips?

Routine 3: Weight-shifting

Here is another way to stay mindful of how weight shifts from the heel through the ball of the foot and toes. You can do this routine anywhere, in shoes or barefoot.

1. Stand in the Power Stance, with your weight on the outsides of your feet and your heels.

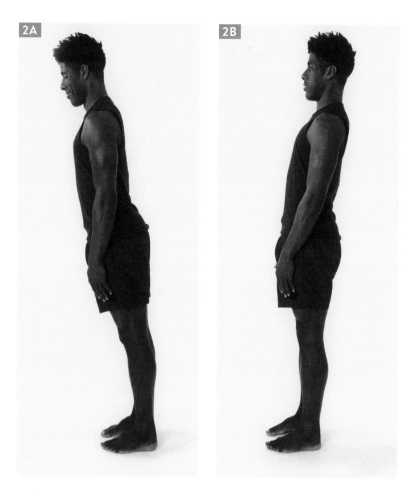

2. Shift your weight to the backs of both heels, then forward through the center of the foot to the balls of the feet and the toes, and back into the back heels. Do this several times.

3. Now shift your weight from the outsides of the heels through the outsides of your feet and then back again. Repeat several times.

4. Finally, shift your weight from the inner sides of your heels through the inside edges of your feet and back, transferring your weight forward and back a few times.

5. Come back to the Power Stance and notice the effects.

TIP You can use this routine as a standing meditation to keep you mindful and develop a habit of transferring your weight correctly when you walk.

FEEL THE EFFECTS

- Have you found parts of your feet that you may not have really noticed before?

- Do you feel it's now possible to transfer your weight from the heels to the balls of the feet to your toes?

- Can you do this along the three separate lines of the foot?

This week you learned two fundamental routines that will be with you for the rest of your life. By doing the Walking Test, you became aware in a totally new way of how you use your feet. You also learned that you can use it to walk your shoes out of your feet. With the Power Stance you learned to lift your arches and keep your feet in a position that fully supports you. You discovered that stepping into the stance makes you feel more active, alive and energetic.

The heel routines taught you to stand solidly on your heels – the first step in creating a fully functional gait. In Week 2, you'll develop what you learned from the Power Stance about the outside edges of your feet by creating movement through them.

WEEK 2:

OUTSIDE EDGE DRILLS

Having learned the Power Stance, you already know how much better it feels to stand on the outside edges of your feet. Still, you'll need lots of practice before you can fully use this part of the foot when you walk.

If you're like most people, you haven't been aware that you don't actually use the outside edges of your feet, so developing an awareness of this and beginning to move in the correct way will be a new experience. To get the best results, I advise summoning up the mindfulness you developed in Week 1.

This week you'll learn specific, focused routines that teach you how to use the outside edge of your foot when you walk. Once you can do this, you'll be putting the greatest weight into the strongest part of your foot.

You'll also begin learning to walk using all the parts of your foot in their natural, logical order, which will prevent your arch and/or big toe from losing their ability to function properly due to excess weight-bearing and repetitive movement.

The routines this week focus on the heel bone, the long bone (the fifth metatarsal) and the bones of the little and fourth toes.

WEEK 2 GUIDELINES

Begin each practice session with the Walking Test. Start each routine with the Power Stance and return to the stance after doing the routine so you can take notice of the effects. Then end with the Walking Test and make a note of any changes you feel.

• DAYS 1–2

Do one of the heel stimulation routines from Week 1 that you felt was most effective. Then do the Outside Edge Walking routine (see p.81).

• DAY 3

Choose a different heel routine from Week 1. Then practice Outside Edge Walking and work on creating length from the outer heel through the side of the little toe.

• DAYS 4–5

Continue with Outside Edge Walking and add Strengthening the Outer Foot (see p.86), along with the heel routine you find the most effective.

• DAY 6

If you feel you've been able to develop some movement along your outside edges, do Advanced Outside Edge Walking (see p.84). If not, continue with Outside Edge Walking. Follow this with Strengthening the Outer Foot and Aligning the Outer Foot with the Hands (see p.88).

• DAY 7

Pick one or two of the routines you already did this week and add Pinky Toe to Outside Heel (see p.92).

Routine 1: Outside Edge Walking

This is a basic routine that everyone can practice to start developing movement in the outside edge of the foot. It's terrific for people who can't place each toe down separately in the Walking Test.

In Outside Edge Walking you walk only with the outside edge of the foot. It forces you to use only this edge and the fifth and fourth toes, and it keeps you off the places in your foot that commonly break down because of overuse. This routine is particularly effective for bunions, plantar fasciitis and dropped arches.

While at first the entire outer foot might feel like a single unit, it's actually possible to lengthen and separate the different parts and move mindfully through them one after another. Once you start being able to do this, move on to Advanced Outside Edge Walking (see p.84). If you aren't ready for the advanced version by the end of this week, don't worry. Eventually, you'll notice you're gaining more and more movement in that area and can begin doing the advanced routine.

1. Create your Power Stance.

2. Step forward with one foot, placing the center heel down, then bring the weight to the outer heel.

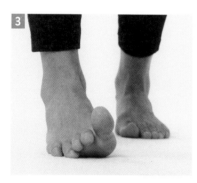

3. Bend your knee on that leg, press all your weight forward on the outer foot, and lower your fourth and fifth toes. Try to press these two toes into the floor.

4. Balancing on the outer edge, bring the other foot forward. Repeat steps 2 and 3 on the second foot.

5. Continue until each foot has taken about ten steps.

6. Return to your Power Stance and notice the effects.

TIPS

- You can practice Outside Edge Walking whenever you're out walking during the day. No one can tell that you're doing it, and it will help you get better at using that outside edge.

- When you're tired and your energy is low, take a few steps using Outside Edge Walking and feel your body and energy level lift.

FEEL THE EFFECTS

- Do you feel that you're standing stronger on the outside edges of your feet?

- Has your weight shifted so that most of it goes into the outer foot, rather than the inner side?

- Are you standing taller?

- Is it harder to collapse down into your feet when you stand on the outside edges?

Routine 2: Advanced Outside Edge Walking

Begin doing this routine instead of the first version once you begin to feel increased length along the outer foot. It will create still more movement through that area. Basically, wherever two bones meet, there should be movement between them, so that as your weight shifts forward through your outer foot, you can reach forward from each bone to the next. Doing this takes concentration and practice but once you get it, you can clearly feel it happening.

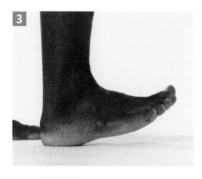

1. Create your Power Stance.

2. Step forward, placing the center of the heel down.

3. Bring your weight into the outer heel.

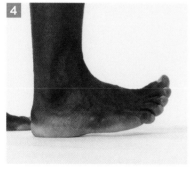

4. Bend your knee and push the outer heel down into the floor. Try to stretch the rest of the outside edge forward: place the long bone down, then the ball of the foot, and finally stretch the little toe forward. This may feel impossible when you first attempt

it, but if you focus on imagining it happening as you work to stretch, eventually it will!

5. Step the back heel forward and repeat step 4 for eight to ten steps with each foot. Your goal is to develop a controlled movement through the outside edges of your feet.

6. Return to the Power Stance and feel the effects.

FEEL THE EFFECTS

- Does it feel easier to stand in your Power Stance at the end of the exercise?

- Do you feel stronger standing on the outer edges of your feet? Does standing this way support your body to be more upright?

- Is it harder for your weight to collapse down into your feet?

- Do your knees and hips feel looser from stretching the outer foot forward? Elongating the outer foot releases the entire outer leg. The knee relaxes, and if it's gripping, it lets go. The same relaxation happens in the hips – and you can feel it.

Routine 3: Strengthening the Outer Foot

This routine develops additional mobility and strength in the outer foot. You need to repeat the action four or five times on each side to feel its invigorating and strengthening effects.

1. Create your Power Stance.

2. Step one foot forward and transfer your weight to the outer heel.

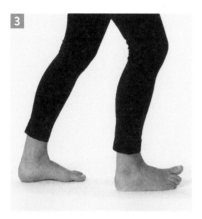

3. Bend your knee and press all your weight into the outer heel, then the entire outer foot. As you do this, keep the outer foot in a straight line. Your outer ankle and knee should line up with the outside edge of the foot.

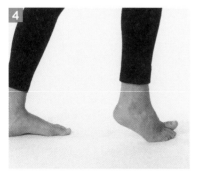

4. Lift your heel and press all your weight into the outer ball of the foot and fifth and fourth toes. Hold for about five seconds.

5. Push the outer ball of the foot into the floor and slowly lower the outer edge to the floor, coming back to the outside heel and then the center heel. As you pull your heel down, make sure it doesn't turn inward but stays in line with the rest of the outer foot. Pulling the heel straight back allows you to feel the lengthening of the outside edge of the foot.

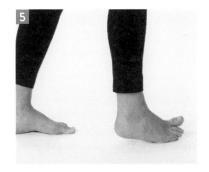

6. Repeat four more times with this foot.

7. Return to your Power Stance and feel the results.

8. Do the same work on your other foot.

FEEL THE EFFECTS

- Do you feel your outer foot planted more solidly on the floor? Does this area feel stronger and more alive?

- Do you feel the outside edges of your feet lifting and supporting your body?

Routine 4: Aligning the Outer Foot with the Hands

Sometimes it's hard to stand on the outer foot because the bones there are not working as they should be. As I explained in Chapter 2, because most people's weight collapses into their feet, the foot bones eventually spread out, lose correct alignment and no longer help support foot function.

In this routine, you use your hands to help set each of those bones on the floor in a straight line, re-educating them about where they're supposed to be. Often the little toe turns in toward the other toes and the long bone splays out to the side. These misalignments throw your weight into the rest of the foot, making it almost impossible to stand strong on the outer foot.

After doing this routine, you'll be standing even taller on the outsides of your feet. You'll feel as though your bones have remembered where they belong and how they're supposed to work. Once you've learned to align them, you can do this routine whenever you notice them falling out of alignment.

Do this routine with your feet on a yoga mat, towel or carpet, since you'll be pressing your foot bones into the floor. If you have difficulty reaching your feet when sitting in a chair, you can do the routine on the floor with your knee bent.

1. Sit in a chair with your feet parallel and in line with your knees.

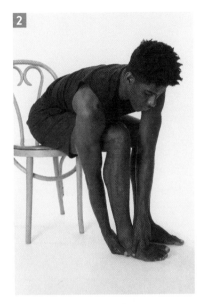

2. Bend forward and turn one foot on its outside edge. With one hand, hold your heel. Slide one finger of the other hand forward between the heel and the floor until you feel a protrusion, which is about two fingers' width from the front of the heel. That is one end of the long bone. Use the hand holding the heel to gently pull the heel backwards and push it down into the floor.

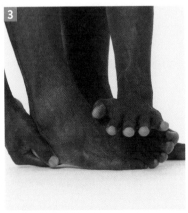

3. Take the hand that found the end of the bone out from under the foot and move it to the inner edge of the foot, right above that protrusion, and use that hand to press the protrusion into the floor. The first hand continues to pull the heel back. Make sure to keep the bone in line with the outer heel. Hold for about ten seconds.

4. The hand holding the heel continues pulling it back. Slide one finger of the other hand out along the long bone toward the pinky toe. Move the hand pressing the protrusion back under the heel and slide one finger out along the long bone toward the pinky toe. Just before the toe you will feel the 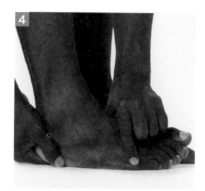 other end of the bone. Move your hand to the inner edge of the foot and press this point into the floor as the other hand pulls the heel back and down.

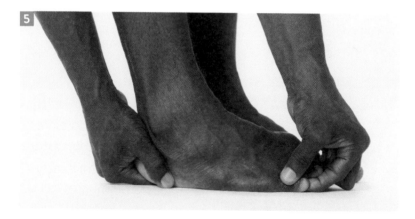

5. Once the entire outer foot is flat on the floor and in a straight line, continue pulling the heel back with one hand. With the other hand grasp the pinky toe, pull it forward, and flatten its side to the floor. Hold both heel and toe, pulling them away from each other and pressing them into the floor for 20 to 25 seconds.

6. Let go of the foot and stand in the Power Stance to feel the effects of waking up these bones.

7. Repeat with the other foot.

TIP Whenever you feel your weight dropping into your inner arches, take time to awaken and align these outer-edge bones and see how quickly your posture improves. This is a mindful, proactive approach.

FEEL THE EFFECTS

- Do you feel the bones in your outer foot pressing firmly into the floor? Are these bones supporting you to stand taller?

- Do they feel more alive, as though they have grasped their purpose of helping you stand stronger and more upright?

- Do you feel that this support prevents your weight from dropping into your inner foot?

- Has your posture improved?

Routine 5: Pinky Toe to Outside Heel

This routine trains you to press each part of the outside foot down, from the toes to the heels, so you can move both forward and backward through each part of the outer foot.

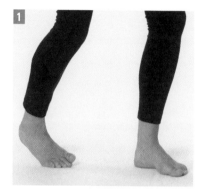

1. Step one foot backward, placing just your pinky and fourth toes and the outside of the ball of the foot down. Bend both knees and press the toes to the floor. Make sure your outer knee stays in line with the outer ankle. The heel can move a bit to the side at first, to help you press just those two toes and the outer ball into the floor.

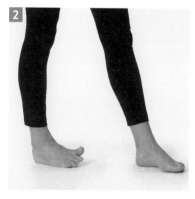

2. Press down and roll backward through the outer ball of the foot all the way to the heel, pulling the outer heel straight back. Your leg will straighten and the weight shift back to your outer heel, then to the center heel.

3. Lift your heel and bring the weight back into the fourth and fifth toes.

4. Repeat steps 2–3 several times.

5. Repeat the whole procedure with the other foot.

6. Return to the Power Stance and feel the effects.

FEEL THE EFFECTS

- Are you standing stronger on the outside edges of your feet?

- Do you feel more balanced as you stand, with your weight neither forward or backward but sitting just in front of your heels?

- Do you feel greater relaxation and ease in your outer feet – as though standing feels lighter and more effortless?

Now you understand how important the outside edges of your feet are for both standing and walking. You've expanded your awareness of how you use your feet to include these outside edges and will be able to use them more mindfully. Just completing Weeks 1 and 2 of the program has given you much more foot awareness and function. So, let's move on to the next step: waking up the balls of your feet.

WEEK 3:

MOVING THROUGH THE BALL OF THE FOOT

Now that you've woken up your heels and begun using your outside edges, you're ready to activate the third part of your feet. This week introduces the ball of the foot, also known as the transverse arch. It's the pivotal point for transferring weight between the heels and toes. In order to transfer weight through the long bones into the toes, there must be a full bend where these bones meet. You must also be able to transfer weight from the outer ball of the foot to the inner ball, and back to the outer ball.

The ball of the foot is well padded to help you roll smoothly through it into the toes. This padding also helps put bounce into your stride as you roll off the ball of the foot into the toes. When you shuffle or slap your feet down, your whole foot moves as one unit instead of transferring weight in sequence from the heel through the ball of the foot into the toes. When you walk mostly using the inside edges of your feet, your weight goes straight from the heel to the big toe, bypassing the ball. These misaligned gaits also send extra pressure into your knees and hips, causing unnecessary wear and tear on those joints.

Many people habitually stand with their weight bearing into the ball of the foot and the toes. Because the ball is squashed into the floor, it can't do

WEEK 3 GUIDELINES

As before, begin each practice session with the Walking Test. Start each routine with the Power Stance and return to the stance after doing the routine to take note of the effects. End with the Walking Test and make a note of any changes.

• DAYS 1–2

Pick one heel routine and one outside edge routine. Practice those then shift back into the Power Stance before doing Waking Up the Ball – Foot Forward (see p.97).

• DAYS 3–4

Do one heel routine and one outside edge routine. You can do the same ones as Days 1 and 2 or choose a different routine in each category. Now is the time to switch to Advanced Outside Edge Walking (see p.84) if you've developed some movement through the outside edges. Shift back into Power Stance and do Waking Up the Ball – Foot Behind (see p.100).

• DAYS 5–7

Do one heel routine and one for the outside edge – the ones you feel will benefit your feet the most. These could be the same ones you did on the previous days or different ones in each category. Follow them with Rolling Through the Whole Ball (see p.103) and Straight Walking (see p.105).

its job of transfering weight, nor can the toes do their job properly. This is why Foot Fix begins by teaching you to stand in your heels. Once you can do this, you understand precisely what it means to transfer weight into the ball of your foot instead of always standing on it.

If this is the first time you've paid attention to the ball of your foot, you'll find that this week's routines will give you a totally new awareness of how critical this part of the foot is. As you roll through the ball of the foot with each step, your body lifts as the weight shifts forward, making it feel much lighter.

Routine 1: Waking up the Ball – Foot Forward

Bending your foot in this routine trains it to roll through the ball into the toes. The more asleep this area has been, the more challenging this action may be for you. Remember that pressing separately into each toe joint wakes up the entire ball of the foot. Pressing strongly down into each joint has the paradoxical effect that when you finish and take the Power Stance, the ball feels lighter, as though it's hardly touching the floor. And you need this lift in order to roll successfully through the ball – you can't do this if it's pressing heavily into the floor.

In this routine, hold onto a tabletop or chair for balance if you need to.

1. Feel steady and mindful in your Power Stance.

2. Step one foot forward. Make sure your feet are parallel and keep them that way during the entire routine.

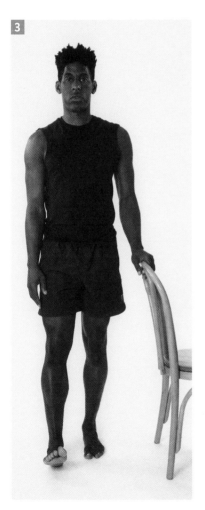

3. Bend both knees slightly and press the center front of the front-foot heel into the floor with the toes and ball of this foot lifted off the floor.

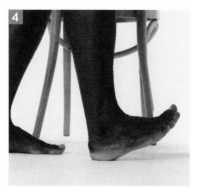

4. Transfer your weight to the outer heel and then through the outer foot to the outer ball of the foot.

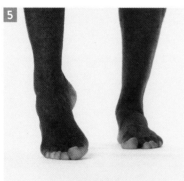

5. Now, lift the heel as high as you can. Shift your weight far enough forward to feel the weight bearing into that outer ball.

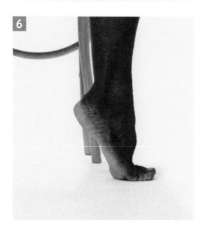

6. Press into the ball at its joint with each toe – the point just below where it meets the toe – starting with the fifth toe, then the fourth, third, second and, finally, big toe. Then reverse direction and press back from the big toe to the fifth.

7. Slowly press backward along the outer foot to the center heel.

8. Repeat steps 2–7 five times, focusing on pressing into the ball at each toe and using all your weight at each one.

9. Step back into the Power Stance and feel the effects.

10. Repeat the routine with the other foot.

TIP Do not let your knee move inward farther than the big toe when pressing into that joint.

FEEL THE EFFECTS

- Does the ball of each foot feel lighter, with less weight bearing into it?

- Do your toes sit more lightly on the floor?

- Where is your weight? More on the heel and outer foot? Is it now easier to transfer weight through the ball of your foot?

Routine 2: Waking up the Ball – Foot Behind

When you walk, both the foot in front and the one behind you must be able to roll through the ball into the toes. This routine is similar to the previous one but trains each foot to shift from the heel into each joint in the ball when the foot is behind you. The more smoothly the ball of the foot can transfer weight, the more easily your movement flows through the muscle chains of the legs.

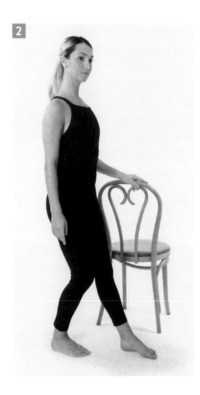

In this routine, hold onto a tabletop or chair for balance if you need to.

1. Step one foot backward. Make sure both feet are parallel and keep them that way during the entire routine.

2. Shift your weight into the entire back foot.

3. Shift your weight to the outer heel.

4. Bend the knee and lift the heel, rolling through the outer foot into the outer ball of the foot. Press all your weight into the outer ball.

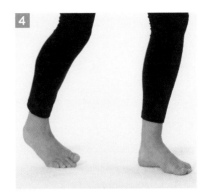

5. Lift the heel as high as you can, then press each ball/toe joint down, from the fifth toe to the big toe. Then, reverse direction and press from the big toe to the fifth.

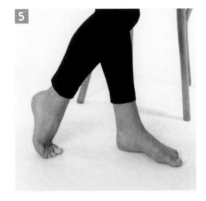

6. Keeping the knees slightly bent, press backward through the outer foot to the outer heel. Place the entire heel down, bringing the body weight into the back foot. Repeat five times.

7. Step into the Power Stance and feel the effects.

8. Repeat with the other foot.

TIPS

- Do not let the knee turn in farther than the big toe.

- Watch that both feet stay parallel.

FEEL THE EFFECTS

- Has your weight shifted more into your heels and outer feet, with much less weight bearing into the ball of the foot and the toes?

- Do you feel generally lighter on your feet?

Routine 3: Rolling Through the Whole Ball of the Foot

Have you noticed that elite runners seem to scarcely touch the ground when they run? I call this style "running up." These runners use the ball of the foot and the toes to propel themselves forward. The ball acts like a springboard, and the body lifts. The torso is completely erect and doesn't lean forward in front of feet as most people's bodies do when they run. You may not be an elite runner, but you're learning here to do what these runners do to make your own stride light and effortless.

This routine focuses on rolling through the entire foot, preparing the feet to practice Straight Walking (see p.105). As you begin to shift your weight into the ball of the foot, you hit the back of the ball then roll through the rest of the ball into the toes. It's important to be able to feel yourself move from the first point to the second point on the ball. You're not just stepping on one point, but creating a rolling action through the full width of the ball. This action then transports you into the toes.

1. Step one foot behind you, making sure your feet are parallel. Lean your body weight into the back leg and foot.

2. Bend both knees slightly, then lift the back heel, bending the back knee more.

3. Lift the heel as high as you can, press the ball of the foot into the floor, and roll through the center of the ball into the toes. Keep both knees bent. This allows you to press all five toes down strongly, letting all your weight bear into the ball as you roll through it.

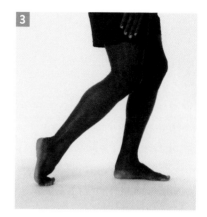

4. Roll backward, pressing from the front to the back of the ball, then pulling the heel back down to the floor and shifting the weight into the back leg. The front knee will straighten.

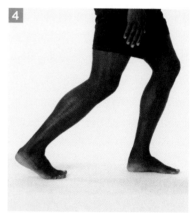

5. Repeat five times, then do the same with the other foot.

6. Come into the Power Stance and notice the effects.

FEEL THE EFFECTS

- As you roll through the ball of each foot, feel your torso lift.

- As you roll into all five toes, feel the power the toes have for keeping the body strong and balanced.

- Does your body feel lighter and more lifted?

- Are you stronger and more balanced on your feet than you were before? Do your hips feel lighter, as if weight has shifted out of them?

Routine 4: Straight Walking – Walking Through the Entire Foot

This routine puts together everything you've learned up to this point. Now that you've woken up the balls of your feet and can mindfully transfer your weight along their entire outside edge, you're ready to learn to walk through the center of your foot using all its parts. This means transferring the weight from the entire heel through the full width of the middle foot and the ball and into all five toes. I call this routine Straight Walking because you're practicing walking straight through each foot. Start out slowly, concentrating on one step at a time. Once you get the hang of it, you can speed up and practice walking at your normal pace.

Rolling through the entire foot releases tension in the lower back. Straight Walking can be tiring at first, because you're training the muscles from your feet all the way up to your hips to work together in a new way. But stick with it and walking will soon become easier!

During the day, you can alternate this routine with the Walking Test to stay as mindful as possible when walking.

1. Bring one foot forward and place the heel, then the ball down, pressing all five toes into the floor.

2. Lift the back heel and roll through the ball of the back foot and into the toes. As you lift the back foot and bring it forward, keep all five toes of the front foot pressed into the floor to help you balance.

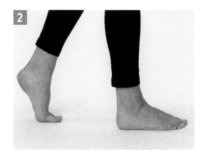

3. Place the heel and ball of what is now the front foot down as you lift the heel of the foot behind you and roll through the ball into the toes.

4. Continue practicing for five minutes, keeping your main focus on the back foot. Be mindful that you are always keeping both feet parallel.

5. Return to the Power Stance and notice the effects.

TIPS

- As you roll through the ball and toes of the back foot, notice how pressing the toes into the floor lifts your body and takes you forward.

- Keep your weight in the center of the foot, making sure you transfer the weight through the full width of the foot and all five toes.

- Know that the more fully you can roll through the balls of your feet, the healthier your leg joints and back will be.

FEEL THE EFFECTS

- Feel how walking this way engages the muscles all the way up the legs to the hips and buttocks.

- Become aware of how your two feet experience Straight Walking differently and require you to focus differently on each foot. We always have one foot that is more challenged and needs more work and attention than the other. If you notice it's harder to roll through the ball and toes on one foot, work more on strengthening and stretching the toes of that foot.

My Left Foot

I myself need to pay much more attention to my left foot to keep it walking properly through all its parts. Even then it gets lazy and sloppy and tires quicker than my right foot. For this reason, I always do more repetitions of a routine with my left foot.

This week you learned to transfer weight through the ball of the foot: from the pinky toe side to the big toe side, and through the entire ball to the toes. Now you've experienced the way this part of the foot is meant to work as part of optimal foot function. The ball of the foot transfers weight into the toes, and in Week 4 you'll discover the last component of a healthy stride – building strength and flexibility in the toes.

WEEK 4:

THE TOES

Did you know that your toes stop functioning as they should when they're stuck in almost all types of shoes? Toes are meant to lift and reach out as you step, then press into the ground and propel you forward. They help you balance when standing and walking.

Sadly, fashionable pointy-toed shoes and other styles with narrow toe boxes cramp the toes into a confined space and eventually distort them. After hours in tight shoes, the muscles in the toes contract, and slowly all the leg muscles become tight and tense as a result.

Since most of us have to wear shoes, it's important to learn how to keep our toes working no matter what style we choose. That's why you need to give some love to your toes when you take your shoes off at the end of the day. Strengthening your toes, moving and stretching them, will get you standing taller, improve your balance and actually boost your energy. You'll feel a connection from your toes all the way through your legs to your hips, and you'll have greater ease of movement through all the joints in between.

WEEK 4 GUIDELINES

As before, begin each practice session with the Walking Test. Start each routine with the Power Stance and return to the stance after doing the routine so you can take notice of the effects. Then end with the Walking Test to see how your gait has improved.

• DAY 1

Choose one heel routine, one outside edge routine and one ball of the foot routine – whichever ones you like and feel are most effective – and practice those. Then do the Seated Toe Stretch (see p.112).

• DAY 2

Repeat Day 1 but this time try the Standing Toe Stretch (see p.113). If you find it difficult, do the seated version again.

• DAYS 3–4

Take the Power Stance, then practice one routine from each of the previous three weeks. You can do the same ones you did on Days 1 and 2 or choose different ones. Then do Stretching and Strengthening Each Toe (see p.115). Remember to stand in the Power Stance afterward to feel the effects. Notice when you end with the Walking Test how much more you're using each part of your feet now your toes are more active.

• DAYS 5–6

Do one heel routine, one outside edge routine, one for the ball of the foot and one toe stretch. Follow this with either Seated Top of Foot Stretch (see p.120) or Standing Top of Foot Stretch (see p.122).

• DAY 7

Repeat Days 5–6 but add Straight Walking from Week 3 (see p.105) to practice rolling through all ten toes as you walk.

The routines for these last three days stretch the muscles that run from just below the knees to the ends of the toes in both the bottom and top of the foot. When both these sets of muscles are working, the toes have optimal function.

The Week 4 Foot Fix routines will teach you to stretch and strengthen your toes, restore their length and realign them correctly. Even if you wear pointy-toed high heels all day, these routines will revive your toes and restore their proper alignment. Just a few minutes of stretching and strengthening will naturally bring your toes back to a healthier position. And once the toes know what it's like to have strength, flexibility and full movement, only two to three minutes of work on them after wearing any type of shoes will quickly restore them, because they now want to feel this way all the time.

Routine 1: Toe Stretch

Seated

1. Sit in a chair with your feet parallel and hip width apart. Slide your feet backward so your heels come off the floor and the balls of your feet press into the floor.

2. Lift your heels as high as you can and press all five toes down with some strength. This will also engage the legs, but it's important that the toes, not the legs, do the work of pressing. Hold for ten seconds, then relax the toes and lower the heels to starting position. Repeat the lifting, pressing and lowering five to six times.

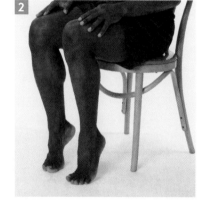

3. Once you can easily press all five toes down, try pressing hard enough to lift onto the tips of the toes. You might not get all toe tips to touch the floor, but you can press the big toe and toes two and three enough to lift the balls of the feet and come up

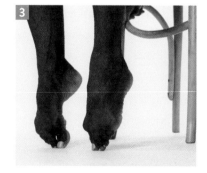

onto those tips. Once you can do this, turn your heels out slightly and try to lift onto the fourth and fifth toe tips.

TIPS

- It's possible to use your leg strength to push into the floor without activating the toes, so be aware of this.

- Repeat the routine more often on the foot that does it less easily.

- Don't worry if your toe bones crack during this routine. It means you're creating more space in the toe joints

---

Standing

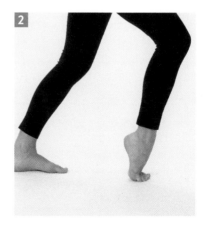

1. Take the Power Stance and step one foot forward.

2. Bend the knee slightly and shift your weight forward into that foot. Lift the heel as high as you can, shifting your weight forward into the toes. Press all five toes into the floor.

3. Slowly lower the heel to the floor, making sure you keep it parallel. Avoid letting the heel move inward.

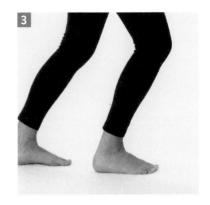

4. Repeat steps 2 and 3 five times, pressing all five toes down as strongly as you can.

5. Repeat on the other foot.

TIPS

- Try to keep the toes straight and flat on the floor when pressing them down. Some toes will want to bend up at the joints.

- Do more repetitions and press the toes down longer with the foot that seems weakest.

- If you have trouble balancing, hold onto a chair back or tabletop.

FEEL THE EFFECTS (FOR BOTH TOE STRETCHES)

- Are you standing taller, with improved posture?

- Do you feel lighter on your feet?

- Do you feel that the toes can lift your body?

Routine 2: Stretching and Strengthening Each Toe

Whenever I teach this routine people immediately exclaim that their eyes are more wide open, their jaws are more relaxed and they feel an immediate sense of general well-being. Because this routine focuses on each toe separately, it stimulates many of the toe reflex points, which connect to the sinuses, eyes and other parts of the head.

I suggest working one foot at a time because working each toe and straightening it out sometimes requires both hands.

1. Sit in a chair with your feet parallel and hip width apart.

2. Bend forward and take hold of the little toe of one foot. Stretch it forward, making it as straight as you can. Keep it straight as you hold it down on the floor.

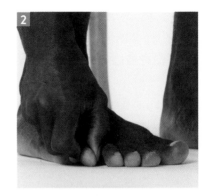

3. Lift the heel as high as you can, using your hands to keep the toe stretched out flat and straight on the floor. Be sure to keep the outside edge of the foot in a straight line from the little toe to the outside edge of the heel.

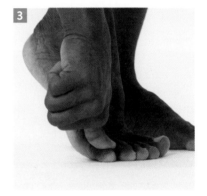

4. Lower the heel, pulling it backward and down to the floor. You should feel a stretch at the little toe if you are pulling the heel backward, not just lowering it to the floor.

5. Repeat steps 2–4 a total of five times, trying to stretch the toe out straighter and longer each time. As you lower the heel, try to pull the toe farther forward. Make sure you pull the heel straight back each time you lower it.

6. Repeat steps 2–5 with the other toes.

7. Before working on the other foot, stand in the Power Stance and feel the effects.

8. After working on both feet, stand in the Power Stance and notice any changes throughout your body.

TIPS

- Try to keep the outside edge of the foot in a straight line as you stretch each toe.

- Keep pulling the heel back as far as it will go as you lower it.

- After each repetition, adjust your grasp on the toe you're working so you can stretch it farther before lifting the heel again.

- If a toe is really twisted, curved or folded under, use both hands to hold it as straight as you can.

FEEL THE EFFECTS

- Do you feel lighter on your feet?

- Do your toes feel longer and more relaxed?

- After you have worked on one foot, does that side of your body feel different? Does the front of the body feel longer and lighter?

- After working on both feet, what differences did you notice between them? Were some toes tighter and more twisted on one foot than the other? Were some toes harder to stretch? Were you unable to keep the outer edge straight as you pulled the heel back? Differences like these show you which parts of each foot you need to focus on.

Stretching the Tops of the Feet

Do you ever think about the top of your foot, as opposed to the sole? Dancers and practitioners of yoga, Pilates, martial arts and other mindful approaches to the body might work the top of the foot, but in general this is a forgotten area, prevented from stretching naturally by our shoes. Many people have no muscle function in the tops of their feet. They can't extend their toes out or stretch through the top of the foot. Yet the foot can't function fully unless the top as well as the bottom is activated. That's why, if you're like most people, you need to stretch the tops of your feet.

When you stretch your toes forward, you're stretching the top of the foot, using muscles called extensors. When you pull your toes up toward you, you're stretching the bottom of the foot, using the flexor muscles. If only one of these sets of muscles is working, the foot can't possibly have its full range of motion. When the tops of the feet are too tight, the toes stay slightly lifted and are unable to press into the floor. When the bottom-foot muscles are too tight, the toes can't extend forward with each step and press down.

This routine takes care of these issues. The first time you do it, you may be shocked to discover how tight this area is. Perhaps you can't bend the top of your foot at all, or it's really stiff and bending it hurts in a way you've never felt before.

Once the top as well as the bottom foot muscles are relaxed, toned and equally activated, you'll find that when you stand, the weight of your torso bears into the neutral point slightly behind the front of the ankle. You'll feel relaxed, with no stress in your feet or body and no excess weight in the toes and ball or the heels. You'll easily shift back into the heels or forward into the toes and ball.

Note: when you first do this routine you might get a cramp in your calves or feet. That happens because this stretch is a new experience for the muscles that run up the leg. It simply means you have woken up an old pattern of tightness in these muscles. After you've done the routine several times, the cramp will be gone. However, if you experienced this routine as very intense, I suggest continuing to do it once or twice a week after completing the program to keep these muscles working well.

This routine has both seated and standing versions. It's usually such a new sensation to stretch the top of the foot that you'll find it easier to start with the seated version. Do one foot at a time if that's more comfortable.

Routine 3: Top of Foot Stretch

Seated

1. Sit in a chair with your feet parallel and hip width apart. Your heels should be directly under your knees.

2. Slide both feet backward so the heels naturally lift off the floor.

3. Lift either one foot at a time or both feet together and tuck the toes under, placing the tops of the feet and toes on the floor. The toes press into the floor. Keep both heels pointing straight back.

4. Press the tops of both feet into the floor and hold for five to ten seconds. You will feel pressure mostly on toes 1–4.

5. Release both feet, then repeat steps 2–4 four more times.

6. Turn your heels out and bring the big toes in toward each other. Press both feet down, angling them so you feel the pressure on the fourth and fifth toes. Hold for five to ten seconds. Release and repeat four more times.

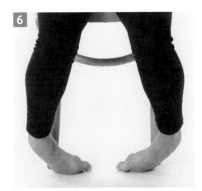

7. Now bring the heels in toward each other so the toes face out. This position allows you to focus on toes 1 and 2. Press them down and hold for five to ten seconds. Release and repeat four more times.

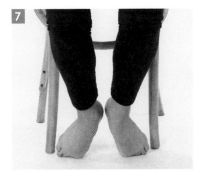

8. Stand up, take the Power Stance and feel the effects in your feet and the rest of your body.

> **TIP** If you find this routine difficult, try working one foot at a time.

Standing

1. Stand in the Power Stance.

2. Step one foot behind you and place the top of the foot on the floor. At first you may only be able to get the very tips of the toes or the toenails on the floor. With practice the tops of your feet will grow more flexible.

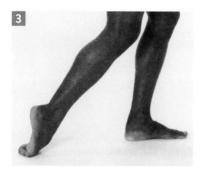

3. Bend both knees. Keeping the foot, ankle, heel and knee in a straight line with the hip, press the top of the back foot into the floor. Hold for five to ten seconds.

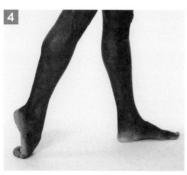

4. Slowly straighten the legs, focusing on straightening the back leg as much as you can. Straightening the legs stretches the top of the foot even more.

5. Repeat steps 2–4 four to five times.

6. To work toes 4 and 5, turn the heel of the back leg out. This position puts more weight into the outer foot. Start with both knees bent, pressing your weight into the outer edge of the back foot. As you straighten the legs, press the back foot down more strongly. Straightening the legs increases the pressure. Hold for five to ten seconds and repeat four to five times.

7. To work the big toe and second toe, turn the back heel in. Bend both knees and press the top of the foot into the floor. Straighten both legs and press harder, increasing the intensity of the stretch in the foot. Hold for five to ten seconds and repeat four to five times.

8. Repeat on the other foot before ending with the Power Stance and noticing the effects.

TIPS

- If this routine is uncomfortable on a bare floor, do it on a mat, folded towel or carpet.

- If it's hard to keep your balance, hold onto a tabletop or chair.

- If one foot is less flexible, hold the pressure longer and do more repetitions of the routines.

- Similarly, if you find any of the positions, such as heel in or heel out, harder to work in, spend a little longer holding those stretches.

FEEL THE EFFECTS (FOR BOTH STRETCHES)

• Does your body weight shift slightly backward?

• Do you feel lighter in your toes?

• Does your whole body feel lighter and more lifted?

Now that you've completed Week 4, you'll realize how essential your toes are to a fully functional stride. Because they get more compressed by shoes than any other part of your feet, I hope you'll want to continue working the toes to restore and maintain their flexibility – from both the bottom and the top.

Once you have worked through all four weeks of the Foot Fix program, I strongly encourage you to continue to exercise your feet on a regular basis. Consistency is key. A daily five-minute foot workout – or even two or three times a week – is all you'll need to prevent your feet from falling back into their old patterns.

The Daily Workout

Here's how to put the four weeks of routines together to create a daily five-minute foot workout.

- Start by using the Walking Test to stay mindful of each part of the foot – it takes only four to five steps to do this.

- Use the Power Stance throughout the day to strengthen the outside edge and activate your toes.

- To create your short practice: choose one heel routine, one outside edge routine, one for the ball of the foot and one for the toes. Start with the ones you like, but be sure to mix things up and add in the routines you found most challenging – your feet need them! If you work on your feet every day, try doing the same four routines for a week, then pick four different ones for the following week.

- Once your feet are pretty well activated, remember to stay mindful of them. At this point you'll know what your weak points are that need a little more attention and will be able to target these areas with specific routines as necessary to keep them in shape.

Foot Fix will make anyone's feet feel better. But if you have come to this book with a specific foot problem, you're likely to need more targeted work to resolve it. The next chapter will show you how.

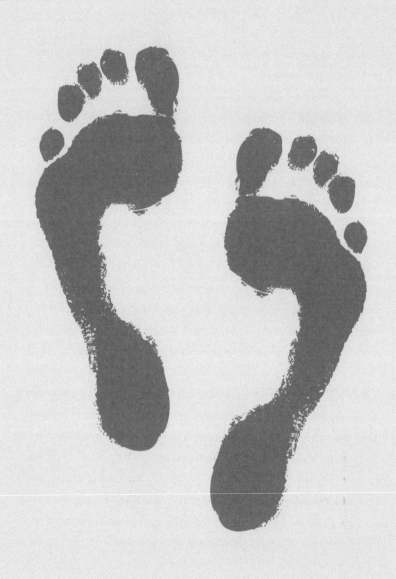

Chapter 4

Common Foot Problems

At the start of every foot class, I ask how many people came because they have foot problems or foot pain. I'm always amazed that out of 40 people, 30 or so will raise their hands. Then I worry that some of them may have serious foot problems that can get worse if they just take a group class rather than a private session where they can be properly assessed and treated. (Since you're working at home alone, I suggest that the moment you feel a sharp pain, stop! Real pain is different from the discomfort that comes from working a part of the body that's never been activated before, and you will know the difference.) But when the class ends, there's always a line of people wanting to speak to me.

And what they say is that just this one-hour group class has created profound changes in their feet and given them personal epiphanies that they just have to share. Sarah, for example, told me she'd had surgery for two bunions several years before and had recently been diagnosed with Morton's neuroma (see p.149). During the class she realized no one had ever told her that the way she walked had caused her bunions. She had no idea that she had to change her gait if she wanted to avoid more foot problems – like Morton's neuroma. Understanding that improving her gait could heal her feet was a real "Aha!" moment. She knew this would require more than one class, but she was confident she'd find her path to do it.

I hear this kind of story often. When people finally discover that the foot problems plaguing them could have been fixed long before, without medical intervention, they feel robbed of possibilities. Yet they're also optimistic, since they know that achieving this awareness is the first step on the way to relieving their pain.

Foot problems are now so common that most people experience them at some point in their lives. In the past, women had the majority of foot problems, and experts blamed high heels and pointy-toed shoes. But today, these problems are prevalent among men as well as women, including people who do a lot of sports. So, the experts began to think the cause might be sports shoes, or other shoes that both men and women wear. My own conviction is that the fundamental reason most foot problems occur is that we have never learned to use our feet fully. Schools don't teach this. Perhaps if they did, we'd have fewer foot, knee and hip problems as we age.

There are many types of foot problems, but for this chapter I have selected six that affect both men and women and are caused either by incorrect gait and posture, certain types of shoes, or both – which means you can relieve them yourself! For each problem, I'll explain what it is and a little about what causes it, before suggesting helpful routines and mindful practices that you can use going forward.

My years of observing and treating people's feet have taught me that the most common foot problems are all caused by walking and standing patterns that send all the weight into the inner sides of the feet. I've labeled these problems according to their familiar medical diagnoses but, in truth, I don't like "name-calling" – in the feet or anywhere else in the body. I believe it is so much more beneficial to understand how your feet got like this than to name the condition. I find that once people clearly grasp this information, they're ready to learn how to self-heal and then maintain a healthy walking pattern.

All foot problems require learning how to use your feet differently so you stop exacerbating your problem. Know that you have the ability to improve your feet no matter what diagnosis you have been given. The problems I cover here can be greatly improved or even reversed. You simply need to put in the effort and then stay mindful of your changed walking pattern. If you fall back into your old pattern, your discomfort will recur. Think of it as a mindfulness bell that snaps your awareness back to your new way of walking and standing.

You need to do the full four-week Foot Fix program as part of fixing any of these problems in order to get the results you want. You'll be pleasantly surprised at how much improvement you'll see just by getting all four parts of the feet fully functional – since their lack of function is what caused the problem in the first place. The specific routines in this chapter will help you to fix your problem once you are familiar with the exercises in the four-week program. All the problems also have "quick fix" routines to help relieve pain. As your understanding of each part of the foot and how they all work together grows, you'll automatically know which parts to work on if you feel discomfort or catch yourself falling back into an unhealthy walking pattern.

BUNION

What it is

A bunion is a bony bump that forms at the joint at the base of the big toe. The enlarged joint sticks out, and the big toe angles in toward the other toes. The joint gets larger due to repetitive weight-bearing over time, and the big toe pushes more into the second toe. The bunion protrudes to the side farther than the big toe used to and eventually calcifies (hardens). The joint can become extremely inflamed and painful, and be hard to bend.

What causes it

While some bunions are apparently caused by inherited factors such as foot structure, many people get them without heredity being involved. In my experience, the misaligned gait that I describe as the heel-to-big-toe gait (see p.42) is the one most responsible for developing a bunion. Every step sends the weight directly into the big toe.

Tight shoes with narrow toe beds are major culprits for this, which seems to explain why many more women than men develop bunions. Stilettos with pointy toes, for example, shift the weight into the ball of the foot and push the big toe in towards the other toes. Women who walk with their knees bent in toward each other and their feet turned out are also at risk of developing bunions, since their weight bears into the balls and toes.

What you need to remember, however, is that whether your bunions are caused by genetics, by your gait or by your shoes, you don't have to live with them!

How to fix it

Bunions are not hard to fix. But you need to support the routines recommended below by physically preventing your big toe from angling toward the other toes whenever you can. Buy a toe separator (see p.177) that creates space between the big toe and second toe and wear it at home and while you sleep.

If your bunion is just beginning, you have a good chance of preventing it from getting worse and even of straightening out the big toe and restoring its natural flexibility and movement. Once the bunion is deeply formed, you can reduce the inflammation, restore the joint's flexibility and stop it from getting any worse. The bunion bump might not completely go away but the pain and discomfort will. In both cases, you'll need to stay mindful and keep checking that you are not falling back into your old patterns.

Follow the protocol below every day for two weeks, while also fitting the Quick Fix into your day. This will retrain your feet out of the pattern that caused the bunion. Once you become mindful enough to no longer walk into your big toe, continue with the Quick Fix and the stretches in Step 5 below at least three times a week to prevent the pattern from recurring over time. Depending on the severity of the bunion, you may need to do this for several months to improve it. Then, to ensure you don't slip back into bad walking habits, continue to practice the Quick Fix and Step 5 stretches once a week.

1. Do the Walking Test (see p.58) to learn which parts of your feet are working as they should be and which parts aren't. Most likely you'll find that you aren't using your outer edges at all but instead are walking with a heel-to-big-toe gait. Perhaps you can't put each toe down separately or roll through each part of the ball of your foot. Perhaps your ankles and knees also drop inward. If you have this pattern, pay attention to what happens to the big toe of the front foot as the back foot comes forward. Is it pushing toward the second toe? Does all your weight bear into it?

2. Use the Power Stance (see p.63) regularly throughout the day to train yourself to stand strong on the outside edges of your feet. Perhaps you can't lower the big and second toes to the floor. Don't worry – as each part of your foot learns to work separately, takes its natural position and develops tone, the toes will lengthen out, strengthen and come down to the floor. The ball of the foot will widen and become able to transfer the weight into all five toes.

3. Pick one heel routine and one outer edge routine and practice them along with the Walking Test and Power Stance. Avoid doing Heel-Ball-Toes (see p.73), however, until your big toe is straight out and no longer angles toward the second toe. Training yourself to walk from your heels along the outside edges will keep your weight off your bunions. As you begin to stand in your heels habitually, you'll develop an awareness of what it feels like to transfer the weight forward through each part of the foot instead of just walking straight into the big toe.

4. Follow these with Waking up the Ball – Foot Forward (see p.97) or Foot Behind (see p.100). This work will train you to transfer your weight from the outside of the ball to the big toe, so you become able to roll through the entire ball of the foot rather than go straight to the big toe.

5. Do the Seated Toe Stretch exercise (see p.112), then Stretching and Strengthening Each Toe (see p.115). Focus intensely on aligning and stretching out each toe at least three to four times per week, to restore the toes' natural alignment and develop their full movement and strength.

Quick fix for bunion

When you're sitting in a chair, cross one leg over the other. With one hand, hold your toe joint firmly just at the bunion. With the other hand, align the toe so it comes straight out from the joint and pull it straight out. Hold it for 15 to 30 seconds, then release. Do this two or three more times. As you stretch the big toe, you can also rotate it clockwise and counterclockwise a little to increase movement in the joint. You can practice this quick fix several times a day.

Mindful practice

When you're standing, consciously shift your weight away from your bunions to the outer edges of your feet and press all ten toes into the floor. Stay mindful during the day and notice when your weight drops into your bunion.

PLANTAR FASCIITIS

What it is

The plantar fascia is a thick band of tough tissue in the sole of the foot that runs from the heel to the base of the toes. When you use your foot in a way that continually places too much stress on the fascia, it can become inflamed and painful. Plantar fasciitis may come on gradually, with mild pain over a period of time, or it may announce itself suddenly with an intense pain that feels like the foot is ripping apart when you get out of bed one morning and try to take a step. In either case the pain usually hits on the inner side of the foot just in front of the heel. When it's really bad it can spread to the outside edge of the foot or the big toe.

What causes it

In the past, plantar fasciitis occurred mostly in pregnant women and overweight people, and experts thought it was due to the extra weight bearing down into the soles of their feet. Today, though, plantar fasciitis knows no boundaries. People with flat feet or high arches and those with diabetes and arthritis also develop it. Another frequent cause is physical activity that strains the fascia, ranging from walking or standing on the job to athletics that can stress the feet, such as running, tennis and high-intensity fitness programs.

People who work out and are in great shape believe that they're immune to developing body problems. Yet they're the ones getting plantar fasciitis in increasing numbers, and doctors are stumped. They're starting to point to the shoes these athletes wear. It's true that these sport shoes are often so soft and cushiony that the feet can just go to sleep in them. Instead of supporting the body, the feet can wind up with little or no muscle tone. It's also true that an inflexible shoe that keeps the foot locked in one position can contribute to plantar fasciitis. However, I don't think blaming shoes is the best path toward fixing the problem.

I've found that in most cases the pain and inflammation occur just in front of the heel on the inside of the foot – exactly the spot where the three long muscles that run down the back of the leg turn under the foot and go toward the toes, helping support the arch and flex the toes. The person's weight collapses right into this point, continually irritating the plantar fascia. The fascia gets stuck to these muscles, preventing them from doing their job of helping transfer weight forward through the foot. Every step tugs on this stuck tissue and irritates it further. In my opinion, plantar fasciitis is never triggered by a single event. It develops over a long period of standing, walking and doing fitness activities with a gait that sends most of the body weight into the inner edge of the foot at that point just in front of the heel.

How to fix it

Plantar fasciitis is easy to address by doing the routines listed here and building the mindful practices into your day.

For two weeks, practice only Steps 1–3 below. Once you can stand on the outsides of your feet, the inflammation should have improved considerably. Follow this by adding in Steps 4 and 5 for a further two weeks. Once you have done this, your pain should be considerably improved. As time passes, it will go away completely, as long as you stay mindful of how you stand and walk.

1. **Do the Walking Test (see p.58) to check your gait.** If you find you can't use your outside edges or place each toe down without letting your knee and ankle move inward farther than the big toe, you know that your walking pattern is a key cause of the plantar fasciitis.

2. **Learn the Power Stance (see p.63) and make it your go-to position** whenever you have to stand for any length of time. Every time your feet hurt, look down, check how you're standing and shift back to the Power Stance. It will give you immediate relief. The Power Stance is probably the most important single action to quickly get out of pain and start healing the inflammation. You can do this essential retraining throughout the day.

3. **Practice Outside Edge Walking (see p.81)** to help lessen the pain and inflammation considerably.

4. **Do Rolling Through the Whole Ball of the Foot (see p.103) and Straight Walking (see p.105),** but begin by rolling just from the outer heel along the outer foot to the ball of the foot, lifting the heel and pressing into the outer ball, then shifting back along the outside edge to the center heel. Do not roll through the entire ball or transfer weight from outer to inner and back again until your pain and inflammation are gone.

5. Work your toes. Once you can stand on your outside edges and work the entire ball of the foot, it's important to align, strengthen and stretch your toes. Do Stretching and Strengthening Each Toe (see p.115) two to three times a week. It's easy to develop strength and flexibility in your toes – and once you practice this last step, your plantar fasciitis will be healed!

6. Be sure to do the mindful practices below as maintenance, to avoid a recurrence of the problem.

Quick fix for plantar fasciitis

The fix here is simply the Power Stance. The moment you feel pain, shift into the stance and it should diminish.

Mindful practices

• Take the Power Stance first thing when you get out of bed, before you walk a step. That way you'll take your first steps of the day with awareness. When we sleep, the body often falls back into old patterns so, to counteract this, take a mindful moment to stand strong.

• When standing during the day, always take the Power Stance to keep your arches lifted and your weight off the painful area. Press all five toes down to activate the muscles along the bottoms of your feet.

- Practice the Walking Test, in shoes or barefoot, to guarantee you aren't walking on your inner edges.

- Only after the pain and inflammation are gone, during both walking and standing, practice rolling from your heels through the entire ball of the foot to all the toes. This is part of retraining yourself to mindfully use your entire foot so you don't fall back into the old pattern.

Rebecca's story

Rebecca woke up one morning and couldn't take a step without excruciating pain. She insisted she had never had foot pain in her life and this just happened without any warning. She went to a doctor who prescribed a boot she was to walk and sleep in. After a month of keeping her foot stuck in this position, the doctor told her to remove it and try to walk without it. It was like learning to walk again, and she was afraid to take a single step. She managed several clumsy steps and felt a slight pain. After her first night without the boot, she got out of bed and tried to stand and the pain was still there. Frustrated, she found her way to me.

Just watching her stand, I knew exactly what the problem was: all her weight was dropping into her inner ankles. I had her try the Walking Test and she could hardly do it. She kept losing her balance. But when I taught her the Power Stance, she felt relief immediately. So I sent her home to practice only the Power Stance. Every time she noticed her feet hurting, she was to look down and see what they were doing. If she wasn't in the Power Stance, she was to go back into it.

She came back the next week with a big smile on her face. In just that week, doing nothing but standing in the Power Stance had relieved her pain and calmed down her inflammation. She was already taking the stance automatically whenever she was standing.

Now Rebecca was ready for the whole program. Each week I chose routines for her – the same routines you'll do in the protocol below – and each week she returned feeling more successful and hungry for more homework. We never got to the fourth week because her plantar fasciitis was healed before then. Although she no longer had pain, she still needed to remain mindful of how she used her feet and she continued doing the routines in the protocol to ensure the problem didn't recur. Rebecca is a great example of what I always tell people: she learned how she created her problem herself, and she fixed it herself.

FALLEN ARCHES AND FLAT FEET

What they are

The sole of a flat foot is completely flat on the floor when you stand. People are often born with flat feet, but they can also develop over time.

Fallen arches are a less severe version of flat feet that develop over years and can eventually become completely flat. If you've been told that you pronate, you're probably developing fallen arches. Fallen arches can cause pain in the feet, ankles, knees, hips or back. Sufferers often say their feet and legs always feel tired. The tired feeling is caused by all the body weight dropping into their legs and feet. That happens because feet with fallen arches can't properly support the body to lift and be upright.

What causes them

When someone is flat-footed from birth, there's usually a genetic link; either a parent or grandparent also has flat feet. People who weren't born with flat feet may develop them later due to an incorrect gait in which all their weight bears down into the inside edges of the feet. The inner ankles drop and the arches slowly collapse (pronation). In particular, someone who walks with their feet turned out and pelvis thrust forward, with their weight going into the inner foot, is more likely to develop fallen arches.

Whether you were born with flat feet or developed them later, you can absolutely turn them around and create healthy arches.

How to fix them

Flat feet and fallen arches aren't difficult to fix, but they require time and persistence. Every step in the Foot Fix program is crucial for you to understand what it takes to build your arches. Once you've successfully done this, consult the points below and choose one or two routines from each of the four Foot Fix weeks – the ones you feel are most effective and that you like best. Continue to do these two or three times a week and remain mindful to avoid slipping back into your old walking pattern.

1. **The Power Stance is key to wake up the outside edges.** Arch building begins with the outside edges of the feet. If you have flat feet or fallen arches, when you first practice the Power Stance, and all your weight is on the outside edges, most of the rest of the foot probably won't touch the floor. This is only to be expected but soon it will start to do so. You'll see your arch beginning to form and your foot function increasing.

2. **The heel routines.** Once you can stand on your heels and feel they are supporting you, use them as a foundation for shifting your weight into the outside edge. Having your heels solid to the ground is the first part of building the arch from the outer foot.

3. **The outside edge routines** develop flexibility and increased movement through the outside edges of your feet. The moment you can stand

on your heels and outside edges, you'll understand why these are the foundations for building your arches.

4. Ball and toe work continues to develop the arches from the outside edges through the entire ball of the foot. Creating movement through the ball is crucial, as the ball and the toes help maintain the lifted arch.

Quick fix for fallen arches

The quick fix here is the Power Stance. Whenever you see yourself falling into the pattern of dropping your arches, switch into the stance. It will immediately remind your feet that lifted arches feel so much better!

Mindful practices

- I can't stress enough the need to stay mindful of your outside edges. Every time you notice your arches dropping, quickly shift back into the Power Stance and remember always to use the entire foot as you walk.

- When in the Power Stance, keep pressing all ten toes into the floor and releasing. Do this all day, whenever you're standing, and feel your arches lift. Strong, engaged toes are key to maintaining healthy arches.

- When you stand or walk, look down every now and then to see where your ankles are. If they're dropping inward, quickly shift into the Power Stance and press the toes into the floor.

HAMMERTOE

What it is

Hammertoe is an abnormal bend in the middle joint of one or more of toes two to four. The joint presses up into your shoe, causing pain and inflammation. Hammertoe can prevent the foot from being comfortable in shoes, but it doesn't always hurt. Over time, though, the joints can harden into the bent position and become more painful. Hammertoe develops slowly, so you might not even realize you have it until you put on narrow or tight shoes or boots and find that they hurt your feet.

What causes it

Hammertoe can be hereditary, but you can still prevent and correct it. Arthritis and diabetes can also cause hammertoe, as can a common gait in which people clench their toes when they walk. This is partly to stabilize and balance themselves but is also a common physical habit people develop out of a general need to feel in control. This gait is a major cause of hammertoe, since when the toes grip, their middle joints bend.

Another cause is a gait that sends the body weight into the inside edges of the feet, pushing the big toe in toward the other toes. This can cause toes to overlap and form hammertoes.

Most often, however, hammertoe is caused by certain types of shoes. Runners often develop the condition, because if their running shoes aren't flexible, the toes can't fully extend forward and are forced to bend up against the front of the toe box. Other kinds of inflexible shoes or shoes that squeeze the toes together also can contribute to forming hammertoe.

How to fix it

Hammertoe is easy to fix if it's just beginning. If it has calcified, however, you need to work on the affected toes regularly every day for two to three minutes. The key to fixing hammertoe is stretching and straightening the muscles on both the bottom and the top of the foot. The more regularly you do this, the quicker you will see results.

First, work through the entire Foot Fix program. Once all the parts of the feet are working, you should see any hammertoes improving as all the toes gain flexibility and become straighter. Then follow the steps below, which are the important focus areas for hammertoes.

1. **Start with the Power Stance (see p.58).** When you stand with your feet parallel and press all your toes into the floor, you are already focusing on your toes, while keeping your feet fully aligned.

2. **Next, work the ball of the foot,** so the toes can stretch out from the joints that connect them to the long bones and begin to straighten. Do Waking Up the Ball – either Foot Forward (see p.97) or Foot Behind

(see p.100) – with three to five repetitions for each foot. Follow this with Rolling Through the Whole Ball of the Foot (see p.103), focusing on Step 3: lifting the back heel, rolling through the ball, and pressing all five toes down. Do this five times with each foot.

This routine helps extend the toes from the bottom of the foot, flattening them out from their joint with the ball. It prepares the foot for toe work. You'll need to add it to your future maintenance routines to prevent the hammertoes from recurring.

3. Now work the toes directly by practicing Seated Toe Stretch (see p.112). As you press the toes down in this routine, focus on lengthening each toe out while keeping it pressed straight down into the floor.

4. Do Stretching and Strengthening Each Toe (see p.115). Use your fingers to press the joint into the floor, and hold it down throughout the routine. Even if the hammertoe has calcified into the bent position, you will be able to straighten it eventually if you keep doing this action.

5. Finish with the Top of Foot Stretch (see p.120). Focus on stretching the muscles that run to the tops of the toes, trying to flatten out each toe. This routine is like ironing out the toe, removing the kink and preventing the joint from calcifying more.

Remember, if you stay proactive and keep stretching and straightening the toes, they'll respond. If you do nothing, they'll get worse – so every bit of time you put toward fixing them counts.

Quick fix for hammertoe

Whenever you think of it, use your hands to stretch and pull each hammertoe out as straight as you can and press it into the floor. Hold it pressed down and extended for 10 to 15 seconds.

Mindful practices

- Whenever you're sitting and can take your shoes off, do the Seated Toe Stretch (see p.112) and Seated Top of Foot Stretch (see p.120) to work on your toes from both sides.

- Whenever you're standing and wearing flexible shoes, do the standing versions of Toe Stretch and Top of Foot Stretch (see p.113 and p.122).

- If you wear high heels with pointy toes, make sure you do a few steps of the Walking Test when you get out of them. Then take five minutes to straighten out and stretch all your toes.

- Whenever you wear shoes that let you move your toes, do keep moving them.

- Practice transferring weight along the ball of the foot from the little toe to the big toe several times a day, so the toes don't stay stuck in one position.

It's Never Too Late

A friend, now in her seventies, who had been a famous model, developed hammertoe. She was convinced the cause was years of having to wear stilettos on the runway. I showed her just the toe routines, and she did them diligently for a year. When I saw her again, she proudly showed me how much straighter her toes were. She couldn't believe her toes could straighten out that much at her age!

MORTON'S NEUROMA

What it is

Developed far more often by women than by men, Morton's neuroma is a swelling of a nerve that leads to a toe. It occurs most often between the third and fourth toes, and sometimes between the second and third toes. The nerve becomes inflamed, causing a painful burning sensation.

What causes it

The main cause of Morton's neuroma is wearing pointed shoes and high heels, which cause the long bones to narrow inward and irritate the nerve. At the same time the padding between the two toes involved starts to wear away. As a result, every step puts pressure into the ball of the foot and this further irritates the nerve. As protection, the nerve develops fluid around it, like a cyst, which becomes inflamed, making every step very painful.

High heels are not the only culprits. Both men and women can develop a neuroma when their shoes are too narrow right at the point where the toes begin. The toes are squeezed toward each other, narrowing the space between the long bones and irritating the nerve.

How to fix it

The essential measure for fixing Morton's neuroma is to remove the pressure from the inflamed area. In most cases the long bones and toes are narrowed in toward each other and need more space between them to allow the inflamed nerve to heal.

If you have this problem, you've most likely been bearing weight into that one point in the ball of the foot for a long time. In order to retrain your feet to keep the weight out of that area, you need to do the entire Foot Fix program. Also, as you begin the program, practice the routine just below every day during the first week. It will start creating space between the long bones and relieve the pressure and inflammation causing your pain. Pay most attention to the space between the two toes where the neuroma is, and hold longer there. Repeat this routine two to three times a day.

1. Place the index finger of either hand between your pinky toe and fourth toe at the base, where the webbing is. Press between the long bones, toward the heel. Try to hold the pressure for 10 to 15 seconds. Keep increasing the pressure to separate the long bones more.

2. Press in the same way between the fourth and third toes, the third and second toes and the second and big toes. Hold for 10 to 15 seconds each time.

3. After working one foot, stand in the Power Stance and see how the toes feel.

4. Repeat with the other foot.

Most likely the area where the neuroma is will be painful at first, but you'll see how quickly it resolves once you give the nerve space to calm down and heal. As you continue with the Foot Fix program, focus particularly on the exercises below. Finally, as you work through Foot Fix, use a toe separator whenever you're at home (see p.177). It will start creating more space between each toe and long bone.

1. The Walking Test (see p.58) will help you figure out exactly what area is taking the most weight. Your goal is to keep the weight off that spot.

2. The Power Stance (see p.63) will enable you to shift the weight onto the outer edges of your feet.

3. The heel routines ground your weight-bearing in your heels – again, away from the affected area in the ball.

4. The outer edge routines encourage your outer foot to effectively transfer weight.

5. The ball of the foot routines help you learn to work each separate point from the little toe side to the big toe side and back again. When you find the painful spot, skip past it and work the areas on both sides. As the entire ball becomes able to work as it was meant to, you'll become adept at shifting your weight away from the point of inflammation, helping the inflammation to subside.

6. **The toe routines** are also critical. Stretching and Strengthening Each Toe (see p.115) creates more space between all the toes and relaxes them. The stretches for the top and bottom of the feet come next, but do these only if they don't hurt. You don't want to cause any more irritation to the inflamed area as you work to heal it! After you've done these routines for a while, see if you can add in one that was too painful when you started.

Quick fix for Morton's neuroma

This is simply to follow steps 1–4 on page 150 whenever your neuroma becomes painful. It will also help prevent a recurrence.

Mindful practices

- When you're wearing shoes that cramp your toes together, be sure not to put weight into the painful area. Mindfully shift through the ball of the foot, transferring your weight away from that area to the outside edge and then to the inside edge. Spend some time on the outside, then shift to the inside edge. Shifting rapidly past the neuroma won't be painful.

- Either when wearing shoes or when barefoot, shift your weight back into your heels to take all the pressure out of the ball of the foot.

- While wearing shoes, keep moving your toes. The more active they are, the less pressure goes into the neuroma.

HALLUX RIGIDUS

What it is

Hallux rigidus simply means "rigid big toe." It occurs when the joint between the long bone and the big toe becomes jammed and can no longer bend without a great deal of pain. The toe slowly stiffens until it's impossible to bend it fully. The joint becomes calcified, arthritic and very thick. It's painful to run or squat, and wearing shoes hurts.

What causes it

Runners and people who play racket sports are prone to developing hallux rigidus. This is because these activities involve aggressive forward thrusting motions with short stops, creating repetitive impact as the big toes jam against the front of shoes and send the impact into the joint. The same thing can happen to long-distance hikers who spend a lot of time walking downhill.

You can also develop hallux rigidus if your regular gait pushes your weight into your big toe, jamming the toe into your shoe and sending impact back into the toe's bottom joint. Eventually, the joint becomes inflamed and calcifies. Still another cause is a hard stub of the big toe. The impact pushes the toe bones back into the joint, and this can develop into hallux rigidus if it isn't treated.

How to fix it

Hallux rigidus can be improved fairly easily if you really work on it when you first notice the toe is bothering you. While trying to bend the joint may be painful, that's exactly what the joint needs in order to recover its full movement! Work just a little each day to create more mobility, then ice the joint or use a topical anti-inflammatory afterwards.

If the big toe is already calcified and the joint can move only with extreme pain, you will experience some pain as you begin to work on it. In that case, apply ice followed by heat, for five to seven minutes each, once or twice a day. A natural anti-inflammatory ointment such as arnica, Traumeel, Zeel or T-Relief will also reduce the swelling. And clay blended with heating and stimulating essential oils, applied thickly, can also pull the swelling out and break down the calcification (see p.172).

Start by following the entire four-week Foot Fix program. This will teach you how to use more of your foot instead of constantly sending impact into the big toe. As you go through the program, focus on the routines and advice described below and also practice the Quick Fix several times a day.

1. **Figure out how you got it.** If you've been practicing any sport or fitness activity that jams your toes against your shoes, pay attention to exactly which moves create the most impact into the big toe. Perhaps you can change the way you step to avoid doing this. There is always a way to alter how you use your feet in order to keep doing what you love.

2. Do the Walking Test (see p.58). If you find that you can't bend through the big toe, pay attention to your gait pattern as you get to that toe. Notice whether you push into the big toe when you're walking barefoot. What exactly does that toe do? Can it extend straight out or does it jam into the irritated joint?

3. Practice the Power Stance (see p.63). When you stand on the outer edges, do your big toes come down to the floor? If not, you know you're bearing weight directly into those toes during all your physical activities and not using your outer edges or heels. Work on the Power Stance so you become able to walk and run on your outer edges while also using all of your toes.

4. Practice Outside Edge Walking (see p.81). Once this is easy to do, switch to Strengthening the Outer Foot (see p.86).

5. Do the ball of the foot routines. To relieve hallux rigidus, you must be able to control where you place your weight on the ball of the foot and toes so that most of the weight doesn't push into the big toe. Start with Waking Up the Ball – Foot Forward or Waking Up the Ball – Foot Behind (see p.97 and p.100). This work enables you to transfer weight from the outside edge to the inside and back again. Once you can do these routines easily, without pain, switch to Rolling Through the Whole Ball of the Foot (see p.103).

6. Do all the toe routines. They will restore movement and strength to all five toes and get them working, so that all your weight doesn't automatically go into the big toe.

Quick fix for hallux rigidus

Do this simple action several times daily. Getting the joint moving as freely as possible will start breaking up the hardened areas and help restore full movement.

1. With the same-side hand, hold the affected joint with the thumb wrapped around the joint at the bottom of the foot while the other fingers hold the big toe from the second-toe side. This keeps the joint correctly aligned.

2. With the other hand, grasp the tip of the toe between thumb, index finger and third finger and push the entire toe directly into the joint. Maintain the pressure for 20 to 30 seconds. Keep increasing the pressure into the toe as you hold it in position.

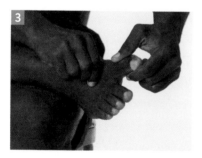

3. Now do the opposite: pull the toe out away from the joint and hold for 15 to 30 seconds. As you stretch the toe out, maintain your grasp on the joint and gently move the toe in circles to increase its movement.

4. Next, see if you can bend the joint a bit.

5. Repeat Steps 2–4 several times each time you do this action. Notice how much more movement you gain each time.

Mindful practices

Using these practices to keep the toe moving and active as much as you can will not harm it. At first you might irritate it slightly, but this will pass as you continue the practices. You'll see increasing movement and decreasing pain within a couple of weeks. If you notice it hurting more or getting inflamed, ice it after working it, or massage an herbal or homeopathic anti-inflammatory product into the joint.

- Avoid whatever activities aggravate the hallux rigidus until the inflammation has decreased and the joint moves easily without pain.

- Stay mindful when you begin doing the activities that caused the problem. Can you shift your weight so it doesn't go into the big toes?

- Practice pressing all five toes down into the floor and releasing them several times a day. Don't let your toes stay passive in your shoes – keep them active!

- Whenever you wear flexible shoes, keep bending your toes by simply lifting your heels as high as you can, then coming down. If doing this hurts the big toe, shift your weight to the outer toes. As your toes become more able to stretch, less pressure will go into the big toe joint.

- When you're wearing shoes, shift your weight through your toes several times a day. Whenever you can take your shoes off, lift your heels and press all five toes into the floor. You want to keep all the toes bending, so the joints stay as flexible as possible.

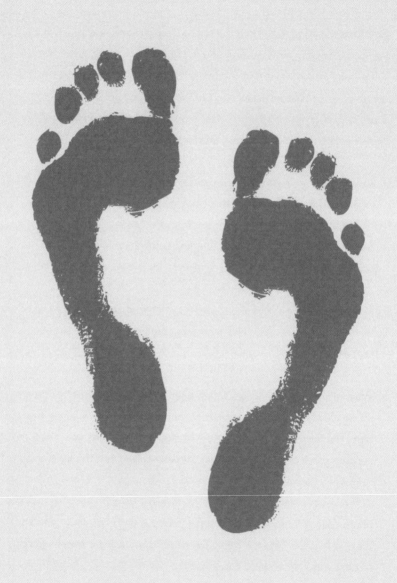

Chapter 5

Maintaining Mindfulness of Your Feet

Once you complete the Foot Fix program, you'll know what it feels like when your feet are doing the job they're designed to do. What's important now is to stay mindful in your feet as much as possible.

One day during the writing of this book, I was standing in my kitchen waiting for the water to boil for a pot of tea and decided to check in with my feet. I looked down and saw that they were exactly parallel to each other. I could feel all their parts activated and supporting me. I had half expected that I'd need to make some corrections, so I was happy to see that they were properly aligned all on their own.

So I wondered: how many times a day could I look down and find them like this? Was I just lucky this time? I decided to make a mental exercise of randomly checking in on my feet when they wouldn't expect it. For the next week, I snuck up on them with quick unexpected check-ins and found that almost every time I was standing much straighter than I had anticipated. Sometimes my left foot was slightly turned out, so I realigned it. But overall my feet no longer fell back into their old patterns as they had in the past.

I realized that because I've been so focused on my feet, and maintained my mindful practices daily for the last two decades, my feet really have shifted into a better way of being. And I promise that if you do the work, your feet, too, will maintain the improvements you create – as long as you stay mindful for a long enough time after completing the program for the changes to really sink in.

No matter what your goal was when you bought this book – perhaps healing a painful condition or keeping your feet healthy to prevent one – foot fitness should be a regular part of your wellness program. In addition to a short daily practice, I encourage you to stay mindful of how you use your feet throughout the day, and to treat yourself to regular foot pampering.

STAYING MINDFUL THROUGH THE DAY

In the previous chapters, I asked you to be mindful of your feet by noticing the effects of the routines when you had completed them. I also gave you mindful practices to do during the day to support the routines. But maintaining this awareness can take other forms. If you incorporate into your day just some of the practices that appeal to you from the following list, you'll find it much easier to maintain your new healthy foot patterns.

First step of the day

Most people roll out of bed in the morning, get to their feet and go. It's automatic. Instead, I urge you to stop, take the Power Stance (see p.58) for a moment, and get grounded in your feet before you take that first step. That first moment you stand up fresh out of bed is crucial. Often feet go back into their old pattern during sleep. Taking that moment to step into the stance gets your mind focused and lines up your body in correct alignment. Standing strong this way not only improves your posture, it gives you more mental clarity by connecting your brain with your body.

Getting focused before taking your first step can also prevent you from hurting yourself, especially as you get older. Often, when older people fall and perhaps break a hip, it happens when they take their first step out of bed in the morning. Pausing for just a moment to get grounded and feel your feet is such a beneficial way to start the day.

A morning Power Stance is also important for anyone with foot problems. Taking that first step mindlessly into a bunion takes you right into the pattern you want to break. If you have plantar fasciitis, taking that first step without first mindfully taking the Power Stance can put you in excruciating pain. Thinking about what you are doing and starting out "on the right foot" will make a big difference.

For anyone, this simple pause can make you more mindful in your body and feet and change the entire way you go through your day.

Morning routine

Once you've taken that pause and stepped into the Power Stance, your brain is already connected to your feet. As you stand at the bathroom sink, you can now actively move your feet and wake them up further by pressing and releasing your toes to build strength and flexibility as you brush your teeth and get ready.

Shoes for the day

Think about the day ahead when you choose shoes. If you'll be spending hours on your feet, wear comfortable shoes that let you shift your weight and wiggle your toes. If you need to wear dressier shoes or high heels, choose the pair that's the most comfortable to walk and stand in. Maybe you can wear comfortable shoes at work and bring heels to change into later. The less time you spend in tight, restrictive shoes the better.

At work

If you work at a desk you're lucky, because you can take your shoes off and do some seated routines. Working your feet boosts circulation and energy, which means you'll be invigorated instead of exhausted after sitting all day. If you don't feel like doing routines, you can increase circulation just by moving your toes and pressing each part of your feet into the floor. If you feel uncomfortable taking your shoes off, you can still wiggle your toes, shift your feet around or point and flex them.

If your job requires spending time on your feet, make sure to keep your toes moving. Shift your weight back into your heels and forward into your toes. Press your toes down into your shoes and release them. Shift your weight from the outsides of the balls of the feet to the insides and back. Check in periodically to make sure you're in the Power Stance. Whenever you walk, try to practice the Walking Test (see p.63). Take advantage of everything Foot Fix has taught you, and use it to keep your feet from getting stuck into the shape of your shoes.

After work

At a cocktail party or any event involving a lot of standing, keep wiggling your toes if your shoes give you enough space to do that. I wear high heels myself, and I can do all the following movements in them. Transfer your weight from your little toes to your big toes several times every few minutes. Shift your weight to your outer foot, then to the center, the inner side, and back to the outer edge. Shift it into your heels, then back to the balls of the feet and toes. Each time you shift into your heels, you'll stand straighter and take pressure off the balls and toes. Take the Power Stance to maintain this posture and stay energized. No one can tell when you're doing any of this, so you won't feel self-conscious. Remember: if you move your feet as much as you can, they won't have time to get stuck and begin hurting.

At the gym

During your workout, don't go on automatic pilot: keep your feet mindfully connected to the rest of your body. On the treadmill, turn your music or the television off from time to time and pay attention to your feet. Keep checking in on them to be sure they stay parallel and that your inner ankles don't collapse. Try walking through the outsides of your feet for a while, then try the Walking Test on the treadmill. This will be hard at first, but the more fully you learn to use your feet, the better your workout will be.

Maybe on some days you just want to be mindless, get on the treadmill and go. Give yourself permission to do that once or twice a week. Pretty soon you'll discover how much better your workout is when you stay mindful in your feet.

Standing in the Power Stance will also improve weight lifting. When every part of both feet is planted solidly into the floor, you have more power up through your body. Weight lifting with collapsed arches or ankles is an injury waiting to happen. So, stand strong if you want to build strength.

Similarly, when doing squats, pay attention to your foot and body alignment. The feet, ankles, knees and hips of both the front and back legs should be lined up.

While you're in your training shoes, keep moving your toes and shifting your weight to all the parts of your feet. Occasionally, try working out barefoot, to give your feet a chance to build strength just as the leg muscles do. Try to add some specific foot routines to your regular workout. And if you're training hard for a particular event, take your shoes off at the end of your workout to walk your shoes out of your feet and fully reconnect your leg muscles to your feet.

In the yoga class

When practicing yoga, pay attention to using your outer feet and keeping your toes activated. In standing poses, find your Power Stance and you'll feel much stronger in every pose.

A collapsed arch in the back foot is a frequent cause of hip injury when practicing Warrior 1 and 2 and Ashtanga sequences. Doing these standing poses and the repetitive Ashtanga movements without a strong base in the feet slowly breaks the hip down because all the weight drops into it. When you bring your new mindfulness and Foot Fix knowledge to your yoga practice, you'll see just how important the feet are in yoga.

Heading home

Going home at the end of the day, often all we think about is getting there and collapsing. It's a time when we tend to disconnect from our bodies. If your trip home involves walking, check in with your feet and walk mindfully. This will take you from being tired to feeling more energized. And if your trip home doesn't involve walking, check in with your feet when you get home – be aware of them as you walk to your door, check in with the Power Stance for a moment as you put your key in the lock. You'll feel more present as you walk inside. Small moments can act as a trigger to remind you to think mindfully about your feet.

At home

When you reach home, take your shoes off and spend five minutes walking them out of your feet with the Walking Test. This will relax your feet, relieve the stress of wearing shoes, and restore proper alignment. If your feet are hurting, you'll experience the magic of the Walking Test when you wake up the next morning and the discomfort is gone.

Any time you're relaxing in a chair – watching TV, reading – sneak in your favorite seated routines. And when you're in the kitchen prepping food or at the stove, where are your feet? The Power Stance will keep your posture upright and you won't get tired when standing and cooking. But if you drop your arches and let all your body weight collapse into your feet, exhaustion will hit you when you sit down to eat. Quickly readjust your feet and feel the difference.

Before bed

If you're trying to break any particular foot pattern, practice the routines for that just before bed. When you reprogram your feet just before you turn in, the old pattern is less likely to sneak back as you sleep.

A final note on walking

We spend so many hours a week on our feet! Try spending some of that time focused on your gait. Even comfortable shoes are likely to prevent your feet from moving fully, so do some barefoot walking when you can. I love practicing the Walking Test for five minutes, then shifting my weight from my heels to the balls of my feet and toes. Then I resume my basic walk. To mix it up, I might walk just through the outsides of my feet. Practicing the different types of walking you learned in the Foot Fix routines will help you catch yourself if you fall into an old pattern.

If walking is your fitness practice, alternate between the Walking Test and walking through the entire ball of the foot into all five toes. Stay mindful of keeping your feet parallel, and be aware of your toes. It's easy to forget to use them when you're in shoes. Most walking shoes have ample toe room so ensure that you press all your toes down every few steps.

Once you've been through the four weeks of Foot Fix and have experienced dramatic improvement, you'll see that beyond the suggestions I listed above, there are an infinite number of ways to remain mindful and enjoy the many benefits of healthy feet.

PAMPERING YOUR FEET

There are so many ways to pamper feet that are tired, achy, swollen or cold! Any of the treats suggested below can soothe and relax your feet and your whole body. But they also have healing effects that go beyond pampering.

Massages, pedicures and reflexology

Wherever I travel, the first thing I do on arrival is look for foot massage spas, which are everywhere in major cities. When you walk for hours in a new city or have just gotten off a long flight, your feet are often swollen and achy, and a foot massage is the perfect solution. A 30- or 60-minute massage relaxes the feet, stimulates the reflex points, and helps you sleep better. But you don't have to have been traveling to need a foot massage! Our feet carry us around all day and deserve a regular massage treat. Book one in for yourself to enjoy the relaxing and energizing benefits.

The soles of the feet contain reflex points that correspond to specific zones of the body. Foot reflexology is an ancient form of massage that uses pressure into these points to stimulate all the parts of the body. A weekly or monthly treatment from a good foot reflexologist will positively affect all your vital organs. You wind up feeling renewed throughout your body, not just in your feet.

TLC at home: foot soaks

Pampering yourself at home is definitely something you should do on a regular basis. Your feet will love that extra attention.

You can buy all sorts of foot soaks, exfoliators and essential oils to relax your feet and prevent and heal swollen feet and ankles, as well as soothing and moisturizing lotions intended especially for the feet and legs. My advice is to try out different brands to see which you like best. Or, better yet, make your own.

Basic foot soak recipe

This is the basic formula for any foot soak. You can use just these three ingredients to relax, increase circulation and decrease swelling and inflammation for tired, achy feet. But you can also add essential oils to increase these effects.

- 1 cup (200g) sea salt
- 1 cup (200g) Epsom salts
- 1 cup (210g) baking soda/bicarbonate of soda

Mix these salts together and put ¼ cup (50g) of the mixture into the container you'll use to soak your feet in. Fill the container with warm to comfortably hot water so the water covers your ankles as well as your feet. Soak for 15–20 minutes. To finish, rinse your feet in clear water, warm or cold as you prefer.

Essential oil foot soak

If you want to include essential oils, use no more than six different oils at a time. Put the salt mixture in a glass or ceramic bowl, add 20 drops of each oil you're using and stir into the salt mixture with a wooden spoon for at least a minute. Over the next 24 hours, stir again for a minute or two at least eight or nine times to prevent the salt from clumping. The salt needs this period of time to fully absorb the oil.

To use, put ¼ cup (50g) of the mixture in your soaking container and fill it with warm to comfortably hot water. The warmer the water, the more the salts penetrate. Soak for 15 to 20 minutes. To finish your soak, rinse your feet in clear water, warm or cold as you prefer.

There are different ways to choose oils. Basically I advise: choose the scents you like! If you want to focus on one goal, such as pain relief, choose all your oils from that category.

RELAXATION OILS	CIRCULATION-BOOSTING OILS	ANTI-INFLAMMATORY, PAIN-RELIEVING OILS
Lavender	Ginger	Camomile
Jasmine	Cypress	Lavender
Ylang-ylang	Eucalyptus	Rosemary
Cedarwood	Coriander	Thyme
Camomile	Juniper	Peppermint
Valerian	Lavender	Clary sage
Sandalwood	Neroli	Sandalwood
		Juniper
		Ginger

Clay treatment

Different types of clay – including green clay, bentonite clay, and white Kaolin clay – also have relaxing and analgesic properties. Clay mixed with anti-inflammatory essential oils and herbs has long been used to reduce pain and inflammation in all joints and works especially well in the feet and ankles. Many types of clay formulas are commercially available. But again, you can make your own.

Basic clay recipe

> 1 cup (200g) of green, bentonite or white Kaolin clay
> ½ cup (120ml) distilled water
> Up to ¼ cup (60ml) olive oil

Stir the water into the clay (not the clay into the water). If the clay absorbs all the water, add a bit more water. Continue adding water until the mixture has a creamy consistency. Let it sit for an hour. If it's gotten firm, add more water until it has that creamy consistency.

Add 1 tablespoon of olive oil and stir. Keep adding oil, one tablespoon at a time (up to ¼ cup / 60ml), until the clay is creamy again and the oil doesn't separate.

To use: with a serving spoon, scoop out as much clay as the spoon will hold and put it on the part of the foot you're treating. With your hand or a wide knife, spread a layer of clay over the area. It should be between an eighth and a quarter of an inch (3–6mm) thick.

To relieve fluid retention at the end of the day, apply the clay and elevate your foot for an hour. If you're only leaving it on for an hour, you can just let it dry. If you're leaving it on longer, wrap paper towel or thin cotton around the clay, then cover with plastic wrap. You can also put a sock on to hold it in place and sleep with it.

An hour is the minimum, but the longer you leave it on, the more therapeutic effects you will get.

Essential oil clay

If you like, you can enhance the properties of the clay by adding essential oils in the same way as for salts. For every cup (200g) of clay, add ten drops of each oil you're using and stir thoroughly to ensure that the oil is thoroughly mixed in.

CBD oil

Research studies indicate that CBD oil can relieve joint pain and inflammation, and there are some CBD products developed specifically for foot pain. In my experience, some people find CBD oil great for reducing pain and inflammation, while for others it does nothing. If you'd like to try it, I suggest doing as much research as you can before choosing a brand and type.

Self-massage

Finally, if you can't get to a spa, try some foot massage on yourself. There are plenty of books and online tutorials on massage but here are some simple guidelines to get you started:

1. Start with your toes. Pull each toe out to stretch it. Gently press all around the top of each toe – this stimulates the reflex points for your sinuses, eyes and face. Put your four fingers in between your five toes, press in toward the base of the toes and hold about 30 seconds. This action sets off a relaxation response through the foot and up the leg.

2. Massage the ball of each foot with the heel of the opposite hand. Move the hand to just in front of the heel and slide the heel of the hand along the sole toward the toes.

3. Using both hands, gently massage the top and bottom of each foot.

To get the full benefits of a massage, you need to use a cream or oil as a lubricant. There are many products available, but you can also make your own.

Massage oil recipe

⅓ cup (80ml) grapeseed oil

⅓ cup (80ml) hazelnut oil

⅓ cup (80ml) melted coconut oil

Combine these oils in a jar and shake well until they're fully blended (or use a blender if you have one).

Add up to six essential oils – no more than six drops of each oil. Don't add extra drops if you use fewer than six oils as this will make the blend too strong.

Staying mindful of your feet and giving yourself regular foot treats are essential for maintaining the benefits you achieved through Foot Fix. Whenever you find yourself disconnected from your feet, pick one of the suggestions in this chapter for checking in with them. If you get in the habit of starting your day grounding yourself in the Power Stance, you'll be in the right mental state to stay mindful all day long. And if you love to pamper yourself at home I encourage you to try some of these recipes and experience the effects of different essential oil blends on your feet.

LAST WORD

You've spent these four weeks waking up the four parts of your feet – and in the process, discovered things about your feet you never knew before. You may have taken your feet for granted, and now you have a new respect for what they do for you – when they work properly.

In each week you've felt an improvement in both your feet and the rest of your body. Now that your feet feel so much better, you need only a little continued work to maintain these changes, because you know what your body needs to be at its best. I hope you continue doing this work and giving your feet the TLC they deserve for the rest of your life. You will see how the benefits multiply over time.

RESOURCES

You might also be interested in devices that support foot health.

Toe Separators

Many companies offer products that help create healthy separation between the toes. If your feet and toes are narrowed in from years of wearing tight shoes, a pair of toe separators will release tension and start to separate the toes and long bones. The Yoga Toes brand offers good toe spacing. I suggest putting them on, then lying down for 15 to 20 minutes to let them begin to relax the feet. You'll feel the feet relax first, then the relaxation moving up through the ankles and calves into the thighs and hips.

Some people walk around wearing toe separators, and others practice yoga with them on. If they feel good and you notice a positive effect from them, add them to your pampering choices. Be aware, though, that once the toe separators have separated your toes back to where they are meant to be, you won't feel the relaxation sensation up through your legs, and you no longer need to wear them regularly. In fact you shouldn't do that, since you don't want your toes to stretch to the point where they no longer line up with their corresponding long bones. That is overstretching, and it causes your toes to lose their strength.

There are special toe separators for bunions that hold the big toe away from the second toe, as well as smaller separators that prevent toes from getting too close or overlapping each other and can be used between the toes that most need the separation. You can find them at pharmacies or specialty shoe stores that focus on foot problems and, of course, online.

Do not buy the soft foam separators used in salons for pedicures since they don't separate the toes enough to make a difference.

Toe separator socks separate the toes slightly. Wearing them regularly will give you a little more toe separation than regular socks or stockings.

Here are some sources:

www.yogatoes.com

www.correctoes.com

www.tootsiescare.com for correcting hammertoes

www.toesox.com

www.zentoes.com for bunions

Yamuna Foot Products

Based on my years of healing foot problems, I've created a set of products that enhance and intensify the work you can do on your feet.

My Yamuna Foot Fitness Kit includes a pair of rounded devices called Foot Wakers and an instructional video as a download or DVD. The focus of the Foot Fitness routines is to increase movement through all the parts of the feet. Because you can mold your foot around them, you can create movement faster.

The Wakers are covered with knobbles, which increase superficial circulation. People tell me that after five minutes on the Wakers they have more energy, and their feet tingle.

The Wakers are also an excellent way for people who are diabetic or have neuropathy to do effective foot work while seated.

Yamuna Save Your Feet is a more advanced program that uses Yamuna Foot Savers, a pair of harder, smaller devices. They come with an instructional video as a DVD or download. I think of the Savers work as the graduate school of my foot education. This very detailed work stimulates and realigns the foot bones and increases toe strength and flexibility. You can place each toe separately on a Saver and align, stretch and strengthen it very precisely. The Savers also target the reflex points in the feet.

The Yamuna Sole Heelers are my newest foot tool. I created them to teach young women how to walk gracefully in stilettos and not hurt their feet, but they turned out to be a terrific way for professional dancers and athletes to keep their feet and ankles strong and prevent career-ending injuries. The Sole Heelers have three height levels to adjust to different feet and needs, with a Foot Saver sitting on top. People report healing plantar fasciitis in one session using them.

Yamuna Foot Soaks

I am also an herbalist, so I developed two recipes for salt baths for your feet:

- To The Bone relieves arthritis and achy bones.

- Muscle Relaxing relaxes muscles, reduces swelling, and boosts circulation in the feet.

All my products are available online at:
yamunausa.com; yamunauk.com; yamunacanada.com;
yamunafinland.com; yamunajapan.com; amazon.com.

Yamuna Foot Fitness classes

I have trained and certified Foot Fitness practitioners in many different countries who offer group classes and private sessions. It is always helpful to have a professional check out your feet to learn how to tweak your foot program for better results. Go to www.yamunausa.com or www. yamunaworld.com to find a certified Yamuna practitioner near you. The practitioners also sell the Yamuna products described above.

You can see some of my videos on Facebook and Instagram: @Yamunabody

INDEX

Acknowledgements

I wanted to write this book for a long time. Then in 2019 I was introduced to Kelly Thompson, then a Watkins editor, by another Watkins author, Swami Saradananda. Kelly loved the idea and was a great help in creating the focus and book proposal. She left Watkins before the writing began, but turned *The Foot Fix* over to Fiona Robertson. With Fiona's incredible support and knowledge, the book became a reality. I want to give huge thanks to everyone at Watkins for being so supportive and great to work with at every step of the process. Also, a big thanks to Kelly and Swami Saradananda.

A very special thanks to Stephanie Golden. Without her this book would have been so much harder to write. Her extensive knowledge of editing and publishing made every step much easier. Her incredible focus on detail is truly remarkable.

I am always grateful to my daughter, Yael Zake Becker, because without her birth and her constant support in the growth of all my work worldwide, this book might never have become a reality.

My mother, Lenore Zake, is responsible for my intense focus on the feet and the importance of keeping them strong and functional as the foundation of the body. It was through watching her that I began developing all my foot education over 20 years ago.

Another special thanks to all the Yamuna practitioners worldwide who get this work out to help more and more people overcome foot problems and understand the importance of maintaining healthy feet. Finally, much gratitude to all the people who have used my foot education and greatly improved their feet. They send me testimonials from all over the world.

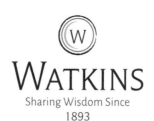

WATKINS

Sharing Wisdom Since
1893

The story of Watkins Publishing dates back to March 1893, when John M. Watkins, a scholar of esotericism, overheard his friend and teacher Madame Blavatsky lamenting the fact that there was nowhere in London to buy books on mysticism, occultism or metaphysics. At that moment Watkins was born, soon to become the home of many of the leading lights of spiritual literature, including Carl Jung, Rudolf Steiner, Alice Bailey and Chögyam Trungpa.

Today our passion for vigorous questioning is still resolute. With over 350 titles on our list, Watkins Publishing reflects the development of spiritual thinking and new science over the past 120 years. We remain at the cutting edge, committed to publishing books that change lives.

DISCOVER MORE ...

Read our blog

Watch and listen to
our authors in action

Sign up to
our mailing list

JOIN IN THE CONVERSATION

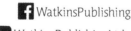 WatkinsPublishing   @watkinswisdom
WatkinsPublishingLtd   +watkinspublishing1893

Our books celebrate conscious, passionate, wise and happy living.
Be part of the community by visiting

www.watkinspublishing.com